ORTHOPEDIC CLINICS OF NORTH AMERICA

www.orthopedic.theclinics.com

Tumors

January 2023 • Volume 54 • Number 1

Editor-in-Chief
FREDERICK M. AZAR

Editorial Board
MICHAEL J. BEEBE
CLAYTON C. BETTIN
TYLER J. BROLIN
JAMES H. CALANDRUCCIO
CHRISTOPHER T. COSGROVE
BENJAMIN J. GREAR
BENJAMIN M. MAUCK
WILLIAM M. MIHALKO
BENJAMIN SHEFFER
KIRK M. THOMPSON
PATRICK C. TOY

ELSEVIER

1600 John F. Kennedy Boulevard • Suite 1800 • Philadelphia, Pennsylvania, 19103-2899.

http://www.orthopedic.theclinics.com

ORTHOPEDIC CLINICS OF NORTH AMERICA Volume 54, Number 1
January 2023 ISSN 0030-5898, ISBN-13: 978-0-323-93883-9

Editor: Megan Ashdown
Developmental Editor: Ann Gielou Posedio

Orthopedic Clinics of North America (ISSN 0030-5898) is published quarterly by Elsevier Inc., 360 Park Avenue South, New York, NY 10010-1710. Months of issue are January, April, July, and October. Business and Editorial Offices: 1600 John F. Kennedy Blvd., Suite 1800, Philadelphia, PA 19103-2899. Customer Service Office: 3251 Riverport Lane, Maryland Heights, MO 63043. Periodicals postage paid at New York, NY and additional mailing offices. Subscription prices are $365.00 per year for (US individuals), $834.00 per year for (US institutions), $433.00 per year (Canadian individuals), $1,019.00 per year (Canadian institutions), $501.00 per year (international individuals), $1,019.00 per year (international institutions), $100.00 per year (US students), $100.00 per year for (Canadian students), $220.00 per year for (international students). Foreign air speed delivery is included in all *Clinics* subscription prices. All prices are subject to change without notice. **POSTMASTER:** Send change of address to *Orthopedic Clinics of North America,* **Elsevier Health Sciences Division, Subscription Customer Service, 3251 Riverport Lane, Maryland Heights, MO 63043. Customer Service (orders, claims, online, change of address): Elsevier Health Sciences Division, Subscription Customer Service, 3251 Riverport Lane, Maryland Heights, MO 63043. Tel: 1-800-654-2452 (U.S. and Canada); 314-447-8871 (outside U.S. and Canada). Fax: 314-447-8029. E-mail:** journalscustomerservice-usa@elsevier.com **(for print support);** journalsonlinesupport-usa@elsevier.com **(for online support).**

Reprints. For copies of 100 or more, of articles in this publication, please contact the Commercial Reprints Department, Elsevier Inc., 360 Park Avenue South, New York, NY 10010-1710. Tel.: 212-633-3874; Fax: 212-633-3820; E-mail: reprints@elsevier.com.

Orthopedic Clinics of North America is covered in *MEDLINE/PubMed (Index Medicus), Cinahl, Excerpta Medica,* and *Cumulative Index to Nursing and Allied Health Literature.*

EDITORIAL BOARD

CONTRIBUTORS

EDITOR

FREDERICK M. AZAR, MD
Chief of Staff, Campbell Clinic, University of
Tennessee Health Science Center, Campbell
Clinic Department of Orthopaedic Surgery
and Biomedical Engineering, Memphis,
Tennessee, USA

AUTHORS

ALEXANDRA M. ARGUELLO, MD
Department of Orthopedic Surgery, Mayo
Clinic, Rochester, Minnesota, USA

ERIC BARCAK, DO
Assistant Professor, Department of
Orthopedic Surgery, John Peter Smith
Hospital, Fort Worth, Texas, USA

JONATHAN D. BARLOW, MD
Associate Professor of Orthopedic Surgery,
Department of Orthopedic Surgery, Mayo
Clinic, Rochester, Minnesota, USA

NICHOLAS BIADASZ, PA-C
Department of Orthopaedic Surgery, Brigham
and Women's Hospital, Boston,
Massachusetts, USA

SARAH R. BLUMENTHAL, MD
Orthopaedic Resident, Department of
Orthopaedic Surgery, University of
Pennsylvania, Philadelphia, Pennsylvania,
USA

DANIEL D. BOHL, MD, MPH
Department of Orthopedic Surgery, Rush
University Medical Center, Chicago, Illinois,
USA

TYLER CALKINS, MD
Orthopaedic Surgery Resident Physician,
Department of Orthopaedic Surgery,
Campbell Clinic Orthopaedics, Memphis,
Tennessee, USA

ANTONIA F. CHEN, MD
Department of Orthopaedic Surgery, Director
of Adult Reconstruction Research, Brigham
and Women's Hospital, Boston,
Massachusetts, USA

ZHONGMING CHEN, MD
Research Fellow, Sinai Hospital of Baltimore,
Rubin Institute for Advanced Orthopedics,
Baltimore, Maryland, USA

CARA A. CIPRIANO, MD, MSc
Chief of the Division of Orthopaedic
Oncology, Associate Professor, Hospital of
the University of Pennsylvania, Philadelphia,
Pennsylvania, USA

THOMAS A. EINHORN, MD, PhD
Emeritus, Department of Orthopaedic
Surgery, NYU Langone Orthopaedic Hospital,
New York, New York, USA

NANCY GIUNTA, PA-C
Department of Orthopaedic Surgery, Brigham
and Women's Hospital, Boston,
Massachusetts, USA

MARCOS R. GONZALEZ, MD
Facultad de Medicina Alberto Hurtado,
Universidad Peruana Cayetano Heredia, Lima,
Peru

ROBERT K. HECK, MD
Professor, Department of Orthopaedic
Surgery, Campbell Clinic Orthopaedics,
Memphis, Tennessee, USA

MATTHEW C. HESS, MD
Department of Orthopaedic Surgery,
University of Alabama-Birmingham,
Birmingham, Alabama, USA

MATTHEW T. HOUDEK, MD
Associate Professor of Orthopedic Surgery,
Fellowship Director, Orthopedic Oncology,
Department of Orthopedic Surgery, Mayo
Clinic, Rochester, Minnesota, USA

EDWARD S. HUR, MD
Department of Orthopedic Surgery, Rush
University Medical Center, Chicago, Illinois,
USA

RICHARD IORIO, MD
Chief, Division of Adult Reconstruction and
Total Joint Replacement, Department of
Orthopaedic Surgery, Brigham and Women's
Hospital, Boston, Massachusetts, USA

LISA KAFCHINSKI, MD
Department of Orthopaedic Surgery,
University of Alabama-Birmingham,
Birmingham, Alabama, USA

RAJ KARIA, MPH
Director of Orthopaedic Research,
Department of Orthopaedic Surgery, NYU
Langone Orthopaedic Hospital, New York,
New York, USA

BILAL KHURSHID, MS
Medical Student, Texas College of
Osteopathic Medicine, Fort Worth, Texas,
USA

JAD LAWAND, MS
Clinical Data Specialist, Spine Surgery,
University of Texas Southwestern, Dallas,
Texas, USA

SIMON LEE, MD
Department of Orthopedic Surgery, Rush
University Medical Center, Chicago, Illinois,
USA

ZACHARY LOEFFELHOLZ, MD
Resident Physician, Department of
Orthopedic Surgery, John Peter Smith
Hospital, Fort Worth, Texas, USA

KENDALL M. MASADA, MD
Orthopaedic Resident, Department of
Orthopaedic Surgery, University of
Pennsylvania, Philadelphia, Pennsylvania, USA

NABIL MEHTA, MD
Department of Orthopedic Surgery, Rush
University Medical Center, Chicago, Illinois,
USA

MICHAEL ALBERT MONT, MD
Orthopaedic Attending, Sinai Hospital of
Baltimore, Rubin Institute for Advanced
Orthopedics, Baltimore, Maryland,
USA

JUAN PRETELL-MAZZINI, MD
Division of Orthopedic Oncology, Chief of
Orthopedic Oncology, Miami Cancer Institute,
Baptist Health System South Florida,
Plantation, Florida, USA

ERIN RANSOM, MD
Department of Orthopaedic Surgery,
University of Alabama-Birmingham,
Birmingham, Alabama, USA

TY K. SUBHAWONG, MD
Department of Radiology, Division of
Musculoskeletal Radiology, University of
Miami Miller School of Medicine, Miami,
Florida, USA

DEVON TOBEY, MD
Orthopaedic Surgery Resident Physician,
Department of Orthopaedic Surgery,
Campbell Clinic Orthopaedics, Memphis,
Tennessee, USA

BENJAMIN K. WILKE, MD
Assistant Professor of Orthopedic Surgery
Mayo Clinic, Department of Orthopedic
Surgery, Mayo Clinic, Jacksonville, Florida,
USA

CLAYTON WING, MD
Orthopaedic Surgery Resident Physician,
Department of Orthopaedic Surgery,
Campbell Clinic Orthopaedics, Memphis,
Tennessee, USA

CONTENTS

Knee and Hip Reconstruction

MyArthritisRx.com (MARx) is an online digital platform with resources to effectively manage osteoarthritis and directs patients to the appropriate information
and tools to manage their disease with or without a coach. The key to self-
management is a self-evaluation and staging program powered by an algorithm based on 150,000 arthritis patients. Outcome data (PROMs), comorbidities, demographics, and personalized characteristics are used to provide a
personalized self-evaluation and staging assessment which characterizes disease severity and risk of progression. The initial 6-week program was
completed by 100 pilot patients with 92% reporting some improvement.
MARx offers evidence of efficacy with promise of cost savings and improved
arthritis care.

Skin antisepsis, such as ready-to-use, no-rinse, 2% chlorhexidine-impregnated
cloths, is one of the fundamental cornerstones for reducing periprosthetic infections after primary lower extremity total joint arthroplasties. This systematic
review presents background material concerning the problem and methods to
deal with and then describes the use of chlorhexidine cloth prophylaxis related
to various surgical applications. The authors found an almost universal benefit
of the cloths. In the meta-analysis, the total pooled effect showed a reduction
in infection rates. The use of chlorhexidine cloths is appropriate for prophylaxis
for knee arthroplasty, hip arthroplasty, and a variety of other surgeries.

With improved chemotherapeutic treatment, patients with primary or metastatic bone tumor have improved prognoses and longer life expectancies; therefore, durable limb-salvage constructs are critical. For tumors of the proximal
femur, endoprosthetic replacement is an option for treatment in primary and
metastatic disease, with the goals being tumor and pain control, earlier mobilization, shorter recovery period, and, in primary tumors, cure. This study provides a summary of current concepts in the treatment of oncologic lesions in
the proximal femur with endoprostheses. Discussion of the inherent complications of these constructs is presented as well as the risks and treatment of
reconstruction failure.

Shoulder and Elbow

The proximal humerus is a common location for primary tumors, benign lesions, and metastatic disease. Advances in neoadjuvant and adjuvant therapy have allowed for limb-salvage surgery in most of the cases. There are numerous of options for surgical management of proximal humerus lesions and the decision to pursue one over another depends on factors such as age, comorbidities, pathology, location within the proximal humerus, planned resection margins/size of defect, and bone quality. Long-term outcomes for these techniques tend to be retrospective comparative studies, with recent studies highlighting the improved outcomes of reverse total shoulders.

Scapular resections are large oncologic undertakings. Due to the soft tissue coverage of the scapula, tumors are often able to be resected with a negative margin. Involvement of the brachial plexus and axillary vessels is rare, allowing for a limb-salvage surgery in most cases. Functional outcomes are based on the magnitude of resection; patients undergoing a partial scapulectomy and those with glenoid preservation demonstrate improved outcomes compared to patients undergoing a total scapulectomy or glenoid resection. Although scapular endoprosthetics are available, there is limited data to support their routine use.

Foot and Ankle

Modern improvements in total ankle arthroplasty (TAA) have increased the performance of this procedure for treatment of end-stage ankle arthritis. A common finding after TAA is the formation of periprosthetic bone cysts, which can be clinically silent or result in TAA failure. The exact cause of periprosthetic bones cysts has not been established, but major theories are related to osteolysis secondary to implant wear, micromotion, and stress shielding. Treatment can be nonoperative with clinical observation for small, asymptomatic cysts. Large, progressive, and symptomatic cysts often merit surgical treatment with debridement and grafting, revision TAA, or salvage arthrodesis.

TUMORS

PREFACE

This issue of *Orthopedic Clinics of North America* is devoted mostly to pathologic conditions of bone, with topics ranging from heterotopic ossification after trauma to oncologic lesions in the upper and lower extremity, as well as those presenting in children. Other topics included are knee arthritis and surgical site infections.

In the upper extremity, the treatment of tumors in the hand and wrist, proximal humerus, and scapula is presented. Giant cell tumor of the distal radius is the topic of discussion in an article by Hess and colleagues. Treatment of this tumor remains challenging because of its high propensity for recurrence and other complications. Often obtaining wide margins to decrease the possibility of local recurrence comes at the expense of optimal wrist function. For primary benign and malignant tumors, the proximal humerus is the most common location. Arguello and colleagues review surgical management options and long-term outcomes, noting improved results after treatment with reverse total shoulder replacement. Unfortunately, endoprosthesis use is not always a possibility for all tumor locations. For scapular tumors, limited outcome data preclude their routine use after resection, although limb salvage surgery is possible in most patients. Scapular tumors require large bone resection, but according to Houdek and colleagues, the brachial plexus and axillary vessels are only infrequently involved, and negative margins are attainable. The best outcomes have been noted in patients with glenoid preservation.

In the lower extremity, Tobey and colleagues discuss the use of joint replacement for the management of bone tumors in the proximal femur. With increased life expectancy, limb-salvage constructions are necessary, with the goals of pain control, early mobilization, shorter recovery, and in primary tumors, cure. Risks, complications, and treatment failures are discussed. When tumors progress to fracture, different fixation strategies are necessary because of impaired bone healing from disease and adjuvant therapies and the higher rates of complications. The fixation principles for pathologic fractures are covered in an article by Masada and colleagues. Concerning fixation and implants, formation of lesions also has been reported after total joint arthroplasty. The exact cause remains unknown, but implant wear, micromotion, and stress shielding are suspected sources. Hur and colleagues describe periprosthetic bone cyst formation after total ankle arthroplasty that can lead to treatment failure. Debridement, grafting, or even revision total ankle arthroplasty may be necessary for large, symptomatic cysts.

Regardless of the anatomic location of tumors, the treatment approach depends on the type of tumor, the risk of progression, symptoms, and stage of, or progression to, malignancy. The same principles are followed in pediatric patients as in adults. Gonzalez and colleagues provide an excellent review of benign bone tumors in children, covering the types of neoplasms, diagnostics, and treatment, which usually is expectant or minimally invasive at first and based on the tumor type, aggressiveness, and likelihood of recurrence.

A common pathologic process after trauma or surgery is heterotopic ossification, which is extra-osseous bone formation in the muscles, soft tissues, and even vascular walls. Some lesions are quite small and clinically insignificant, but others progress to restrict motion and even ankylosis. Lawand and colleagues note that symptoms usually begin 1 to 2 weeks after the inciting event and include erythema, swelling, pain, loss of motion, and joint tenderness. Their article provides an overview of the pathophysiology, epidemiology, prophylaxis, and treatment of postoperative heterotopic ossification.

Another topic of pathology for which a cure remains elusive is osteoarthritis. Many treatment modalities exist to alleviate pain and slow progress, but often joint replacement remains the only end-stage option. Ioria and colleagues developed a digital platform for patients to self-manage their knee arthritis. The program allows patients to self-evaluate and stage their arthritis, characterizing disease severity and risk of progression. The program then directs them to appropriate information and tools to manage their disease. The authors report that 92% of the patients had some improvement during their 6-week pilot program.

Orthop Clin N Am 54 (2023) xi–xii
https://doi.org/10.1016/j.ocl.2022.10.001
0030-5898/23/© 2022 Published by Elsevier Inc.

Surgical site infection remains an important topic of concern for all surgical disciplines. Infection is still a significant cause of morbidity and mortality after surgery. In a meta-analysis and systematic review, Chen and Mont provide the latest information of surgical site infection in total hip arthroplasty, examining the utility of chlorhexidine cloth use for prevention. They found an almost universal benefit and reduction in infection rate in total hip arthroplasty with the use of ready-to-use chlorhexidine cloths after surgery.

I believe this issue will provide our readers with essential information and updates on pathologic conditions of bone and would like to thank the authors for their in-depth reviews on these important topics.

Frederick M. Azar, MD
University of Tennessee Health Science Center
Campbell Clinic Department of Orthopaedic
Surgery and Biomedical Engineering
Memphis, Tennessee 38104, USA

Campbell Clinic Foundation
1211 Union Avenue, Suite 510
Memphis, TN 38104.

E-mail address:
fazar@campbellclinic.com

Knee and Hip Reconstruction

A Digital Platform for the Self-Management of Knee Arthritis: MyArthritisRx.com

Richard Iorio, MD[a,*], Nicholas Biadasz, PA-C[b],
Nancy Giunta, PA-C[b], Antonia F. Chen, MD[b],
Thomas A. Einhorn, MD, PhD[c], Raj Karia, MPH[c]

KEYWORDS

- Conservative arthritis care • Self-management • Digital platform
- Personalized arthritis treatment • Optimization • Staging • Self-evaluation • Arthritis coach

KEY POINTS

- There is no comprehensive digital resource available with the purpose of improving patients' knowledge of their arthritis disease process and treatment options while facilitating the conservative management of their osteoarthritis in a social environment.
- As the COVID-19 pandemic taught us, there is a need for digital tools and resources in the telehealth era. Self-management tools are effective methods for conservative osteoarthritis management.
- Patients can be empowered to choose their arthritis treatment regimen and access a social environment/platform which facilitates contact with providers and other patients.
- The social nature of MyArthritisRx.com(MARx) serves to reduce their feelings of isolation and promote motivational interaction.
- The MARx pilot study offers evidence of efficacy with the promise of cost savings and improved arthritis care.

INTRODUCTION

There is no comprehensive digital resource available with the purpose of improving patients' knowledge of their arthritis disease process and treatment options while facilitating the conservative management of their osteoarthritis in a social environment. As the COVID-19 pandemic taught us, there is a need for digital tools and resources in the telehealth era. Self-management tools are effective methods for conservative osteoarthritis management.[1]

Self-efficacy is considered a core component in self-management. Self-efficacy is a personal judgment of how well one can execute courses of action required to deal with chronic processes. However, there is a lack of knowledge about the association between self-efficacy and health-related outcomes in osteoarthritis. Self-efficacy programs for arthritis need to be incorporated into a digital format.[2–4]

The Centers for Disease Control (CDC) recommends several proven approaches to reduce arthritis pain including a self-management education program, such as the general "Chronic Disease Self-Management Program," which teaches the skills and confidence to live well with arthritis every day.[2] They also recommend physical activity programs that can improve health for participants with arthritis. Walking,

[a] Division of Adult Reconstruction and Total Joint Replacement, Department of Orthopaedic Surgery, Brigham and Women's Hospital, 75 Francis Street, Boston, MA 02115, USA; [b] Department of Orthopaedic Surgery, Brigham and Women's Hospital, 75 Francis Street, Boston, MA 02115, USA; [c] Department of Orthopaedic Surgery, NYU Langone Orthopaedic Hospital, 301 East 17th Street, Suite 1402, New York, NY 10016, USA
* Corresponding author.
E-mail address: riorio@bwh.harvard.edu

Orthop Clin N Am 54 (2023) 1–6
https://doi.org/10.1016/j.ocl.2022.08.005
0030-5898/23/© 2022 Elsevier Inc. All rights reserved.

bicycling, and swimming decrease arthritis pain and improve function, mood, and quality of life.[1]

Non-pharmacological clinical practice guidelines for osteoarthritis include self-management and education, exercise, weight loss if overweight, and joint replacement where appropriate. Some of these elements have been incorporated into programs in the recent past. Patient education, in the form of a supported self-management program, designed to meet these guidelines, has been developed and implemented nationwide through the "Better Management of Patients with Osteoarthritis" program in Sweden. The analog program is based on theories of behavioral change and aims to provide patients with a sense of self-control and knowledge to adopt a healthy and active lifestyle. A total of 3266 patients with hip or knee osteoarthritis participated in this observational, registry-based study. Self-efficacy was assessed using the Arthritis Self-Efficacy Scale. Pain was estimated by self-reporting the number of days per week the patients were physically active $\geq$ 30 min. Results were self-reported at baseline and after 3 and 12 months. High versus low self-efficacy for pain management at baseline resulted in reduced pain and increased physical activity at all follow-ups.[3] High self-efficacy for management of other symptoms resulted in lower pain and higher physical activity at follow-up for pain and physical activity.[4–6] Patients with obesity reported lower activity levels at follow-up as expected.[7]

Developed by a team of researchers at Stanford University, the Arthritis Self-Management Program (ASMP) is a small group, analog education program. It aims to help people with arthritis adapt to their condition and gain confidence and control over their lives. The 6-week course consists of weekly 2 to 2$^{1}/_{2}$ hour interactive workshops in which participants learn and practice techniques for building an arthritis self-management program specific to their needs. Workshops include educational sessions and group discussions to help participants get feedback and suggestions from one another about approaching arthritis-related problems. After each workshop, participants practice recommended approaches on their own and report their progress to the group. The ASMP was highly effective but analog and depend on workshops led by physical therapists.[8]

With increasing prevalence, new arthritis management strategies must be developed to augment the conservative management of arthritis and transition from the analog to the digital age. The use of information technology (IT) resources, including Web-based platforms, mobile applications, and telemedicine, has demonstrated positive results and a growing demand.

Emerging IT platforms can be used to optimize communication between patients and caregivers in novel ways that can improve outcomes. Patients may be able to identify their symptoms early on, and through self-help and exercise programs, gain control over their disease process and postpone surgery and total joint replacement.[9]

HISTORY

MyArthritisRx.com (MARx) is a digital self-management program for osteoarthritis that delivers patient education, targeted exercises, and peer-engagement through a social environment while being supported by arthritis coaches. Numerous studies and focus groups have evaluated this type of tool and found that Web-based education provides a higher level of knowledge retention versus face-to-face interactions, with evidence for self-management success as patients feel as if they can guide their own treatments with some direction from a reliable digital source. The MARx platform has also been targeted toward underserved populations who have not been participatory in the analog programs. Studies have shown the lower rates of seeking Internet health information among Hispanic versus non-Hispanic whites; efforts to increase the use of Internet health resources will help empower patients to self-manage their chronic disease conditions such as arthritis.[10,11]

The MARx digital tool seeks to modernize treatment and control system costs and to improve overall patient outcomes and increases access to care. The Website is designed to educate patients about osteoarthritis (OA) and to differentiate diverse OA phenotypes using fingerprints of arthritic disease. The objective of the MARx project is to identify patients for whom nonoperative management strategies are appropriate to conserve health care resources, improve the health status of individuals and populations, and optimize surgical outcomes when arthroplasty is indicated. The purpose of this observational study is to provide some preliminary results for a digital self-management program for knee osteoarthritis: MARx.

BACKGROUND

MARx provides a comprehensive network of online resources to effectively manage osteoarthritis and directs patients to the appropriate information and tools to manage their disease.

The key to self-management is a self-evaluation and staging program powered by an algorithm based on 150,000 arthritis patents. Outcome data Patient Reported Outcom Measures (PROMs), comorbidities, demographics, and personalized characteristics are used to provide a personalized self-evaluation and staging assessment which defines disease severity and risk of progression.

MARx was developed using a three-tiered Patient-Centered Outcomes Research Institute Grant at New York University Langone Orthopedic Hospital. The authors hosted three focus groups consisting of 10 patients each with a diagnosis of OA, the aim of which was to understand patient goals and perspectives concerning conservative arthritis management. Inclusion criteria included male and female participants ages 18 and older. Questionnaires were distributed to patients inquiring about comorbidities, surgical procedures related to OA, medical management of OA, and satisfaction with current management. In addition, patients were asked to describe their current level of OA understanding, the resources that they use to educate themselves regarding their disease process, and which educational modality (in-person, books, Internet, and television) they preferred. A brief question-and-answer session was included at the end of all sessions. Reviewing their results, the authors found that most patients do not currently use online or Internet-based IT programs to help cope with their osteoarthritis but are interested in trying one (Fig. 1).

The authors' findings also revealed that most patients are more interested in a community program for managing their osteoarthritis than in a computer-based program, but most were interested in some type of self-management program as part of their therapy (Fig. 2). Most patients were interested in a social framework where they could discuss their disease and treatment options with health care professionals and other patients to tailor treatment to their specific needs and lifestyles. Furthermore, there was a sense of dissatisfaction with the current treatment options available to patients; most of the patients interviewed were either neutral or not satisfied with the quality of the treatment they were currently receiving within the health care system (Fig. 3). Last, the authors found patients rely on both themselves and their physician equally when planning their treatment of OA (Fig. 4). Taking these results into consideration, patients desire to be part of a larger community of OA patients, and many believe that they can guide their own treatment regimens with some direction from a reliable source. The patients believed that the current resources available to them were inadequate for their individual needs. The need for shared decision-making tools was obvious to the patients and the caregivers who participated in the focus groups.

There is an initial 6-week program that includes:

- Targeted interactive education modules
- Physical therapy exercise s
- Pain coping strategies and interventions
- Peer interaction for better engagement and support
- A group or personalized arthritis coach or a self-directed program

A long-term maintenance program which is in development includes:

- Access to a social support network of similarly affected users
- Access to online modules and resources
- Quarterly self-assessments
- Arthritis coach support

We report here on our first 100 patients who completed the program.

RESULTS

Forty-two patients participated in the MARx 6-week program; 95% reported improvement in the functional outcome assessment, sit-to-stand test (STS), 55% reported greater than 20% improvement in STS if they completed week 3, and there was a 19% average improvement in the Knee Injury and Osteoarthritis Outcome Score (KOOS) pain score. Most patients (71%) thought empowered to choose their treatment regimen and access a social environment/platform which facilitated contact with providers and other patients. The social nature of MARx served to reduce their feelings of isolation and promote motivational interaction.

TESTIMONIALS

1. "The program was outstanding in many ways. First, I now feel stronger and have less knee pain in my everyday life. Second, I actually liked doing this exercise program; it was well tailored to seniors, though I think it would work well for any age group. It was especially good because of its focus on improving muscle strength for walking and increasing core strength, the latter of which I find the most difficult to accomplish. The exercises are varied by week, in intensity,

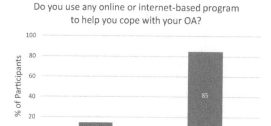

Fig. 1. Would you have interest in an online or Internet-based osteoarthritis management program?[9]

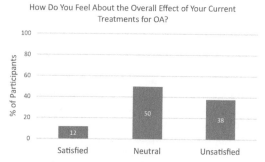

Fig. 3. What are your overall feelings toward current osteoarthritis treatments?[9]

and in difficulty. With some exercises I was a beginner and others I was more advanced. By the end, many of the initially challenging exercises became much easier for me."

2. "Your program is appreciated for giving me those exercises. They encouraged me to keep my circulation going. The exercises helped strengthen the muscles around my arthritic knee making it easier to get around."

3. "I was pleased with the personal touch of the program. I had access to a fitness trainer who monitored my progress and answered my questions. I completed questionnaires about pain levels and progress, which helped the trainer guide me. There were helpful short s on knee replacement topics, medications, and so forth. I found them all very useful. Unlike most other online fitness programs, this one was based on a two-way interaction, and it was motivating to have someone actively following my progress."

DISCUSSION AND SUMMARY

Osteoarthritis is the number one cause of disability in the United States and is the fourth leading cause of hospital stays in the United States. The CDC projects are an increase from 54M US adults affected to 78M by 2040. An arthritis-attributable effect, including arthritis-attributable activity limitations and arthritis-attributable work limitations, and severe joint pain were noted in 20% of those. Estimated annual direct medical costs are at least $140 billion. Sixty percent of Americans with arthritis are of working age (18–64). Eight million working-age adults report inability to work due to arthritis.[9,10] The MARx pilot study offers evidence of efficacy of nonoperative osteoarthritis treatment, with the potential of cost savings and improved arthritis care in this patient population.

The quality of materials available to both patients and physicians in the digital world is of variable quality and reliability. Wiechmann and colleagues[12] examined the quality of smartphone applications available in the iTunes App Store being marketed to health care professionals. With over 20,000 applications in the medical category, the search was narrowed to 7699 applications based on appropriate search criteria (using phrases such as critical care, orthopedics, procedures, and emergency medicine). After reviewing the categories, 64.9% of the applications were not relevant to medical professionals who were referring patients to these applications.[12] It is critical to understand and evaluate specific technologies before using them in one's practice and especially before recommending them to other physicians or patients.[8]

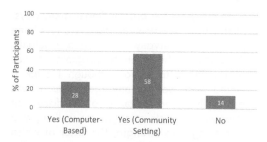

Fig. 2. Would you have interest in an osteoarthritis self-management program?[9]

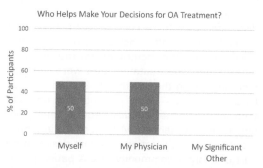

Fig. 4. Who is responsible for your osteoarthritis management?[9]

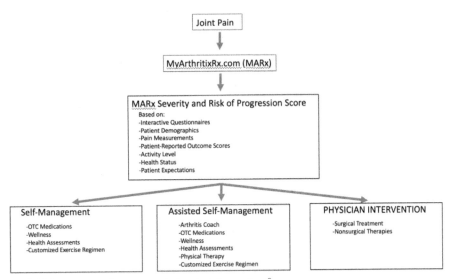

Fig. 5. MyArthritisRx program from presentation to intervention.[9]

Using technology to provide nonoperative osteoarthritis care may reduce health disparities. Health disparities and barriers are faced by minorities when trying to access health care and navigate the health care system, in particular the Latinx population. Unnecessary utilization of medical resources occurs when patients experience barriers to primary care which may include a lack of educational tools for self-directed care. In a CDC analysis of the National Health Interview Survey for 2002, 2003, 2006, and 2009 combined, an estimated 3.1 million Hispanics were noted to have arthritis.[10,11]

The benefit of the MARx platform is that all patients, including underserved patients, are provided with a comprehensive network of resources to effectively manage their osteoarthritis, providing direct value to the patient while decreasing unnecessary resource utilization. Self-management education programs are among the proven approaches to reduce arthritis pain and increase physical activity. This has also been shown in non-English speaking patients, as Web-based platforms are more easily converted to multilingual platforms.[10,11] Payer savings by surgical delay and medication discontinuation are estimated to be $109.1 M/y in a sample of 28,000 arthritis participants in a population of 100,000 captured lives. For 9661 participants with knee osteoarthritis, 966 delayed surgery ($59.2 M saved) and 1430 discontinued medications ($4.2 M saved). In addition, in 6981 participants with hip osteoarthritis, 698 delayed surgery ($41.5 M saved) and 1424 discontinued medications ($4.2 M saved).[9]

The expectation is that the MARx platform could improve patient satisfaction and outcomes through improved accountability, empowerment, and engagement. The ability to connect within the digital community, to use an online arthritis coach and to connect with an advisor to guide the use of digital resources, removes the feelings of isolation and provides the sense of belonging to a larger "arthritis community." System costs will improve by reducing unnecessary utilization of resources such as emergency department visits, unnecessary specialty visits or "no show" appointments, in addition to decreased medication and imaging costs. The projected savings of delayed total joint arthroplasty and decreased visit costs for specialists and therapists in insured populations have been extremely positive, and further studies on the utility of the MARx platform will need to be conducted to validate this. The utility of MARx and other self-management tools in captured populations such as an accountable care organization, Medicare advantage beneficiaries, arthritis longitudinal bundle participants, and the expanded Medicaid population nationally (involving a disproportionate share of underserved populations) is promising.

The MARx program provides a structured exercise program and an easy-access, evidence-based information source. The technology platform includes progress tracking, self-monitoring and coaching as required, and a social media component (in development). Participants are encouraged to take responsibility for those behavioral patterns that influence the OA disease process. The objective of the tools that MARx provides is to engage participants in a social platform and improve compliance with their recommended intervention regimens, increasing mobility, satisfaction, and adherence while decreasing pain scores (**Fig. 5**).

Emerging IT platforms can be used to optimize communication between patients and caregivers in novel ways that can improve outcomes. The MARx platform is designed to engage patients and help patients understand the value of conservative measures to relieve pain and improve health status. Future patients are expected to be better equipped to adapt to a changing health care landscape that will use newer IT resources for self-managed therapies. Properly curated, Web-based education platforms can provide a useful source of evidence-based, standardized patient education. Physicians who treat arthritis should consider how the availability of these IT tools can help provide the best management strategies for their patients, but it is important that all new platforms be properly evaluated before introducing them to patients.

CLINICS CARE POINTS

- There is no comprehensive digital resource available with the purpose of improving patients' knowledge of their arthritis disease process and treatment options while facilitating the conservative management of their osteoarthritis in a social environment.

- With increasing prevalence, new arthritis management strategies must be developed to augment the conservative management of arthritis and transition from the analog to the digital age.

- The MyArthritisRx.com (MARx) program provides a structured exercise program, and an easy-access, evidence-based information source.

- The technology platform includes progress tracking, self-monitoring and coaching as required, and a social media component (in development).

- MARx provides participants with a social platform and improves compliance with their recommended intervention regimens, increasing mobility, satisfaction, and adherence while decreasing pain scores

DISCLOSURE

This work was initially funded by PCORI. myarthritisrx.com, PCORI Tier III (3411628-003) award funding for Lifetime Initiative for the Management of Arthritis studies.

REFERENCES

1. American Academy of Orthopaedic Surgeons Management of Osteoarthritis of the Knee (NonArthroplasty) Evidence-Based Clinical Practice Guideline. Available at: https://www.aaos.org/oak3cpg Published 08/31/2021.

2. Lorig KR, Sobel DS, Ritter PL, et al. Effect of a self-management program on patients with chronic disease. Eff Clin Pract 2001;4:256–62.

3. Thorstensson CA, Garellick G, Rystedt H, et al. Better Management of Patients with osteoarthritis: development and Nationwide implementation of an evidence-based supported osteoarthritis self-management Programme. Musculoskelet Care 2015;13(2):67–75.

4. Degerstedt Å, Hassan A, Thorstensson CA, et al. High self-efficacy – a predictor of reduced pain and higher levels of physical activity among patients with osteoarthritis: an observational study. BMC Musculoskelet Disord 2020;21. 380.

5. Heikkinen K, Helena LK, Tain N, et al. A comparison of two educational interventions for the cognitive empowerment of ambulatory orthopaedic surgery patients. Patient Educ Couns 2008;73(2):272–9.

6. Heikkinen K, Leino-Kilpi H, Salantera S. Ambulatory orthopaedic surgery patients' knowledge with internet-based education. Methods Inf Med 2012; 51(4):295–300.

7. Lee FI, Lee TD, So WK. Effects of a tailor-made exercise program on exercise adherence and health outcomes in patients with knee osteoarthritis: a mixed-methods pilot study. Clin Interv Aging 2016;11:1391–402.

8. Lorig K. The arthritis self-help workshop, leader's manual (revised). Palo Alto (CA): Stanford University Arthritis Center; 2001.

9. Einhorn TA, Osmani FA, Sayeed Y, et al. The role of patient education in arthritis management. The utility of technology. Orthop Clin North Am 2018; 49:389–96.

10. Centers for Disease Control and Prevention (CDC). Prevalence of doctor-diagnosed arthritis and arthritis-attributable effects among Hispanic adults, by Hispanic subgroup–United States, 2002, 2003, 2006, and 2009. MMWR Morb Mortal Wkly Rep 2011;60(6):167–71.

11. Peña-Purcell N. Hispanics' use of Internet health information: an exploratory study. J Med Libr Assoc 2008;96(2):101–7.

12. Wiechmann W, Kwan D, Bokarius A, et al. There's an app for that? Highlighting the difficulty in finding clinically relevant smartphone applications. West J Emerg Med 2016;17(2):191–4.

The Utility of Chlorhexidine Cloth Use for the Prevention of Surgical Site Infections in Total Hip Arthroplasty and Surgical as well as Basic Science Applications

A Meta-Analysis and Systematic Review

Zhongming Chen, MD, Michael Albert Mont, MD*

KEYWORDS

• Infection • Prevention • Total joint arthroplasty • Chlorhexidine cloth • Outcomes

KEY POINTS

- Skin antisepsis is one of the fundamental cornerstones for reducing infections of primary lower extremity total joint arthroplasties.
- Found an almost universal benefit of the ready-to-use, no-rinse, 2% chlorhexidine-impregnated cloths.
- Applies to various surgical applications, such as total knee and hip arthroplasty as well as other surgical specialties.
- Recommend that dual application with use the night before and the morning of surgery should be the standard of care.

INTRODUCTION

The United States has the highest annual reported number of primary lower extremity total joint arthroplasties, with more than 658,000 performed.[1-3] Although knee and hip arthroplasties are highly successful elective surgical procedures with greater than 95% survivorship at 10-year mean follow-ups, there are still estimated to be approximately 80,000 revision procedures performed each year, with the most common reason now being periprosthetic infections.[2-6] Despite the prevention efforts, the infection rates in total knee and hip arthroplasty (TKA and THA) remain at approximately 1.5% or higher.[7,8] Their approximate cost is $75,000

per year per infection,[9] making it close to a $2 billion or more annual problem.

Despite substantial infection prevention efforts, there are reports that demonstrate that the incidence of infection has been increasing.[2,10] Springer and colleagues studied infection among knee and hip arthroplasties[11] in six national arthroplasty registries (ie, American Joint Replacement Registry, Australian Orthopedic Association National Joint Replacement Registry, National Joint Registry of England, Wales, Northern Ireland, and the Isle of Man, New Zealand Joint Registry, Swedish Hip Arthroplasty Register, and the Swedish Knee Arthroplasty Register). Between 2010 and 2015, the incidence of periprosthetic infections

Sinai Hospital of Baltimore, Rubin Institute for Advanced Orthopedics, 2401 West Belvedere Ave, Baltimore, MD 21215, USA
* Corresponding author.
E-mail address: rhondamont@aol.com

Orthop Clin N Am 54 (2023) 7–22
https://doi.org/10.1016/j.ocl.2022.08.004

increased for both knee (0.88%–1.03%) and hip arthroplasty (0.79%–0.97%). Thus, it is imperative that new or improving strategies to reduce infections continue to be advanced.

Surgical site infections (SSIs) are affected by the density of microbes that may contaminate wounds during operations.[12] The endogenous flora of patients' skin is the most common cause of SSIs.[13,14] Although it takes as little as 100 microbes per gram of soft tissue to cause infections, the natural density on the skin may be as great as 2×10^6 bacteria per square centimeter.[13–16] Therefore, prevention protocols implemented for decreasing microorganisms on the skin should decrease rates of SSIs.[3]

There are a multitude of preoperative skin preparation methodologies currently available.[3] One method is ready-to-use, disposable, 2% chlorhexidine-impregnated cloths. These are quick and simple to apply. They only need to be wiped on, and the antiseptic solution rapidly dries without having to be rinsed off. It has been demonstrated that skin treated in this manner retains antimicrobial activity for approximately 6 hours.[17]

Therefore, a basic overview and analysis of antiseptic disinfectants and chlorhexidine cloths is warranted. The authors first describe a comparison of chlorhexidine to other antiseptics and then a comparison of the cloths to solutions. This will then be followed by the main purpose of this study, which is a systematic review of chlorhexidine cloth applications in: (1) surgically relevant basic science studies; (2) knee arthroplasties; (3) hip arthroplasties; and (4) other surgical specialties. In addition, a meta-analysis of the qualifying knee and hip arthroplasty reports will be performed.

This summary of all surgeries will include every report on chlorhexidine cloth applications in TKAs. Although it is expected that TKAs and THAs cannot always be separated in studies, this thorough review will be valuable to knee surgeons.

COMPARISON TO OTHER ANTISEPTICS

Chlorhexidine has been shown to be effective as an antiseptic agent.[18,19] It is a broad-spectrum bactericidal antimicrobial agent with activity against gram-positive and gram-negative bacteria. The mechanism of action is that the chlorhexidine salts dissociate and release cationic ions. These cations bind to the negatively charged bacterial cell walls, disrupting cell membrane integrity and lipid formation, and at high concentrations are bactericidal.[20,21]

The Association of Registered Nurses recommends that patients receive preoperative scrubbing or antiseptic wash the night before or on the day of surgery. The Department of Health and Human Services recommends using an appropriate antiseptic agent for skin preparation and approved the use of preoperative showering or bathing with agents such as chlorhexidine.[12] Kapadia and colleagues investigated the incidence of SSIs in THA patients who used chlorhexidine cloths preoperatively compared with patients who did not.[18] Through a review of their institution's database, 557 patients who used the cloths and 1901 patients who did not use the cloth were studied. They found that a statistically significant lower incidence of infections occurred in patients who were cleaned with cloths (0.5%) when compared with patients who were not (1.7%) at approximately 1 year follow-up ($P = .04$), thus demonstrating the efficacy of chlorhexidine (Fig. 1). Darouiche and colleagues studied whether chlorhexidine and alcohol were superior to povidone-iodine in patients undergoing clean-contaminated surgery (ie, colorectal, small intestinal, gastroesophageal, biliary, thoracic, gynecologic, or urologic operations performed under controlled conditions without substantial spillage or unusual contamination).[22] A total of 849 patients (409 in the chlorhexidine–alcohol group and 440 in the povidone–iodine group) from six hospitals were analyzed. Their outcome of interest was any SSIs within approximately 30 days after surgery and they found that the rate was significantly lower in the chlorhexidine–alcohol group than in the povidone–iodine group (9.5 vs 16.1%; $P = .004$). Thus, this study further suggests the superiority of chlorhexidine compared with povidone-iodine.

ADVANTAGES OF CHLORHEXIDINE CLOTH APPLICATION VERSUS SOLUTIONS

Although there are many studies supporting the efficacy of preoperative chlorhexidine, there are two different ways to dispense the product.[23–30] It can be applied as a solution or in no-rinse impregnated polyester cloth. Edmiston and colleagues supported the efficacy of showering with the solution, but also noted that the cloths might be a superior option.[17] They studied the effect of chlorhexidine solution showering on skin surface concentrations. In a randomized prospective study conducted at a single institution, they analyzed 120 subjects. All of these participants were equally randomized into two groups, two applications (at night and then in

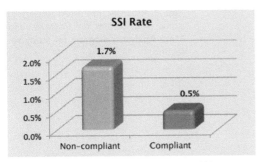

Fig. 1. Surgical site infection (SSI) rates within approximately 1 year follow-up in total hip arthroplasty patients who used chlorhexidine preoperatively (compliant) compared with patients who did not (non-complaint).

the morning), or three applications (two consecutive nights and then in the morning). Each of these groups was also equally subdivided into groups that paused for 0, 1, or 2 minutes before rinsing. Their outcome of measure was chlorhexidine skin surface concentration at approximately 4 hours after the morning application. They found that the mean chlorhexidine concentrations were significantly higher in the 1- and 2-min pause groups compared with the no-pause group in participants taking 2 (978.8 ± 234.6, 1,042.2 ± 219.9, and 265.6 ± 113.3 μg/mL, respectively) or 3 (1,067.2 ± 205.6, 1,017.9 ± 227.8, and 387.1 ± 217.5 μg/mL, respectively) showers ($P < 0.001$). They also investigated the activity of 2% chlorhexidine impregnated preoperative skin preparation cloth compared with an application of 4% chlorhexidine solution.[17] They studied 30 subjects by randomizing their right and left inguinal skin sites into either cloth or solution treatment, respectively. They demonstrated that microbial reduction was significantly greater for the sites treated with the cloths at approximately 10 minutes, 30 minutes, and 6 hours after preparation ($P < 0.01$). The log(10) reductions for cloth-prepped sites at 10 minutes, 30 minutes, and 6 hours were 2.50, 2.33, and 2.54 for the abdominal sites as well as 3.45, 3.50, and 3.64 for the inguinal sites, respectively. However, the log(10) reductions for solution-prepped sites at 10 minutes, 30 minutes, and 6 hours were 2.18, 2.19, and 2.77 for the abdominal sites as well as 2.78, 2.63, and 3.15 for the inguinal sites, respectively. Therefore, this suggested that the cloth application is more advantageous than the solution. There are also many other potential advantages of the cloth application in addition to its superior efficacy compared with solution, such as ease of use and consistent dosing. There

is also no need to rinse it off after usage. As noted in the above study, if the chlorhexidine solution is left on to dry, antimicrobial activity is sustained for approximately 6 hours.[17] In the following review, the authors specifically focus on the use of chlorhexidine cloths and not solutions.

METHODS

A literature search of the PubMed, EMBASE, and Cochrane Library was performed to identify studies evaluating the outcomes of chlorhexidine cloth use in surgeries. Search terms included "chlorhexidine," "gluconate," "wipe," "cloth," "antimicrobial," "antiseptic," "surgery," "hip," and "knee." An exhaustive review of the literature was further generated by looking at the reference list of the found articles.

Our initial search returned a total of 790 records. The products—cloths and solutions—were then clearly delineated. Inclusion criteria included: studies in English language, studies with greater than five cases, and articles reporting on the results of chlorhexidine cloths. Studies reporting only on the outcomes of chlorhexidine solutions were excluded. Other exclusion criteria included: narrative reviews, case reports of individual patients, and series with less than five total patients.

Studies were analyzed regarding their level of evidence. They were classified into: level of evidence I (high-quality prospective cohort studies with adequate power or systematic reviews or meta-analyses of these studies); II (lesser quality prospective cohort studies, retrospective cohort studies, untreated controls from randomized control studies, or systematic reviews of these studies); III (case—control studies or systematic reviews of these studies); IV (case series); and V (expert opinions, unpublished abstracts, case reports or clinical examples, or evidence based on physiology, bench research, or "first principles").[31]

After applying our criteria, 26 studies were deemed eligible and included in our review (Fig. 2).

Eligible knee and hip articles underwent a full-text systematic review of relevant outcome parameters with the primary outcome of interest (decreased rates of infection) coded as a binary variable (decreased vs not decreased). Demographics and infection rates stratified by patient risk were also tabulated. The tabulated results were stratified by surgically relevant basic science studies, TKAs, THAs, and other surgical specialties.

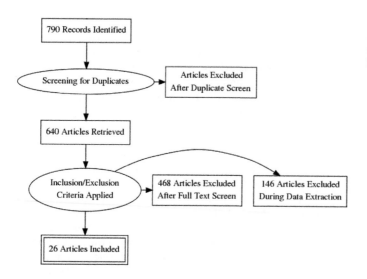

Fig. 2. PRISMA (Preferred Reporting Items for Systematic Reviews and Meta-Analyses) diagram for study selection.

A further meta-analysis was performed to qualify relevant lower extremity joint arthroplasty studies from the above list. The inclusion criteria for the meta-analysis included: studies in English language, those with greater than five cases, and articles reporting on the comparison results of dual application chlorhexidine cloths on lower extremity total joint arthroplasties.

Data were extracted, compiled in a database, and analyzed using Microsoft Excel (Microsoft Corporation, Redmond, WA).

RESULTS
Surgically Relevant Basic Science Studies

A total of seven articles (one level of evidence I and six level of evidence II studies), detailed below, studied chlorhexidine cloth effectiveness from a basic science standpoint.

Edmiston and colleagues studied the superiority of chlorhexidine cloths compared with solution when they investigated the activity of 2% chlorhexidine-impregnated preoperative skin preparation cloth compared with an application of 4% chlorhexidine solution[17] as described in detail above. They demonstrated that the antibacterial effect was greater for the sites treated with the cloths. When it is left on to dry, its antimicrobial activity persists for approximately 6 hours.

A study by Ryder investigated whether 2% no-rinse chlorhexidine cloths improved antiseptic persistence on patients' skin compared with 4% chlorhexidine rinse-off solutions.[32] A total of 24 subjects were equally randomized (level of evidence II) into groups that either used the applications just the morning of the test or the night before and the morning of the test. Testing of the different methods occurred 1 week apart. The outcome of interest was chlorhexidine residual 3 hours after the morning application. The results showed that in both groups, the 2% chlorhexidine cloth subjects had more residual chlorhexidine on their skin than the 4% chlorhexidine solution subjects. Two applications of the 2% chlorhexidine cloth showed more residual chlorhexidine than one (P = 0.016).

Rhee and colleagues investigated whether no-rinse 2% chlorhexidine-impregnated polyester cloth skin application yields greater residual chlorhexidine concentrations and lower bacterial densities on skin versus non-antiseptic cloths or cotton washcloths.[33] In a level of evidence II evidence prospective, randomized 2-center study, 63 participants (126 forearms) received chlorhexidine cloth skin cleansing on 1 forearm, whereas 33 participants received a non-antiseptic-impregnated cellulose/polyester cloth application on the contralateral forearm, and 30 participants were washed with a cotton washcloth dampened with sterile water. Immediately and 6 hours after application, chlorhexidine cloths yielded the highest residual chlorhexidine concentrations (2,500 and 1,250 μg/mL, respectively) and significantly lower bacterial densities compared with non-antiseptic cloths or cotton washcloths (P < 0.001).

Makhni and colleagues prospectively analyzed the effectiveness of chlorhexidine gluconate cloths for decreasing bacterial counts of patients on their posterior neck region.[34] There were 16 healthy adults who participated, where their right side of their neck was wiped twice (ie, the night before and the morning of the experiment) with chlorhexidine gluconate cloths and the left side was used as a control region. Their outcomes of interest were bacterial growth at baseline on enrollment in the study, then on arrival at the hospital, and finally, after both sides of the neck had received standard preoperative scrubbing. All patients had positive bacterial growth at baseline (median > 1000 colonies/mL). When chlorhexidine gluconate cloths were used, bacterial counts were noted to be decreased (mean decrease in bacterial counts was 536 colonies for control and the mean decrease was 790 colonies for the intervention group) before the preoperative scrub, but this finding was not statistically significant ($P = 0.059$). All patients (100%) had no bacteria identified on either side of their neck after completion of the preoperative scrub. Thus, the authors suggested that at-home use of chlorhexidine gluconate cloths may not decrease the topical bacterial burden. However, their results suggested a decrease in bacterial counts with chlorhexidine cloth use, and its insignificance may have been due to the study being underpowered because there were only 16 participants.

Edmiston and colleagues performed a larger study to determine the skin concentrations of chlorhexidine after preoperative showering/skin cleansing using 4% soap compared with application via 2% impregnated polyester cloths.[35] A total of 60 participants were equally randomized into three groups: evening application only; morning application only; or evening and morning after application (level of evidence II). All groups showered with the soap first before a 1-week wash period before applying with the cloths. Their outcomes of interest were chlorhexidine skin surface concentrations at five selected skin sites (right/left antecubital fossa, right/left popliteal fossa, and abdomen) the morning after their respective applications. They found that the chlorhexidine cloths yielded significantly higher skin concentrations of the antiseptic as the mean values ranged from 12.7 to 27.4 times higher in that arm of the study compared with the antiseptic soap group ($P < 0.0001$). Thus, this study further supported the superiority of chlorhexidine cloths compared with solutions.

Whitman and colleagues evaluated the impact of 2% chlorhexidine-impregnated cloths on methicillin-resistant *Staphylococcus aureus* (MRSA) colonization.[36] In a randomized, double-blind, controlled trial, they studied 1,562 US Marine Corps recruits (level of evidence I). A total of 781 were randomized into

the chlorhexidine cloth group and 781 into the control cloth group. Subjects applied their respective cloths three times weekly, with the outcome of interest being the incidence of MRSA colonization during a minimum 6-week follow-up. Their results demonstrated that 77 subjects (4.9%) acquired MRSA and there were significantly fewer in the chlorhexidine group, 26 (3.3%), compared with 51 (6.5%) in the control group ($P = 0.004$).

Edmiston and colleagues investigated the benefit of an electronic alert system for enhancing compliance of preadmission application of 2% chlorhexidine gluconate and the effect of five applications on concentration levels.[37] A total of 100 participants from a single institution were equally randomized to five skin application groups: 1, 2, 3, 4, or 5 consecutive applications (level of evidence II). Subsequently, participants were also further equally randomized into two subgroups: with or without an electronic alert. Their outcome of interest was chlorhexidine skin-surface concentration measured approximately 10 days after final application. They found that the mean composite skin surface chlorhexidine concentrations in participants receiving electronic alerts following 1, 2, 3, 4, and 5 applications were: 1,040.5, 1,334.4, 1,278.2, 1,643.9, and 1,803.1 μg/mL, respectively, whereas composite skin surface concentrations in the no-electronic alert group were: 913.8, 1,240.0, 1,249.8, 1,194.4, and 1,364.2 μg/mL, respectively ($P < 0.001$). Therefore, this demonstrated the efficacy of electronic alerts and patient compliance as well as the sequential increase in chlorhexidine skin concentration with each additional application.

In summary, six of seven basic science articles (level of evidence I, 1 study, level of evidence II, five studies) demonstrated the positive antibacterial results of chlorhexidine cloths (Table 1). Although one other level of evidence II study only trended toward decreased bacterial counts with chlorhexidine cloth use ($P = 0.059$), the insignificant result was possibly due to its low power.

Knee Arthroplasty
The following section evaluates the outcomes of "TKA" using chlorhexidine cloths. In some articles, results combined TKAs and THAs where they could not be separated, and the data will be presented in this section. There were a total of 10 studies, 2 were level of evidence I reports, 6 were level of evidence II, and 2 were unpublished lower level studies (Table 2).

Table 1
Results of basic science reports

Report	Subjects	Results
Edmiston, et al[17] 2007	30	Microbial reduction was significantly greater for the sites treated with the cloths at approximately 10 min, 30 min, and 6 h after preparation ($P < 0.01$)
Ryder,[32] 2007	24	Chlorhexidine cloth subjects had more residual chlorhexidine on their skin than the 4% chlorhexidine solution subjects
Edmiston, et al[35] 2008	60	Chlorhexidine cloths yielded significantly higher skin concentrations (mean values ranged from 12.7 to 27.4 times higher) compared with the antiseptic soap group ($P < 0.0001$)
Whitman, et al[36] 2012	1,562	Significantly less MRSA colonization in the chlorhexidine group, 26 (3.3%), compared with 51 (6.5%) in the control group ($P = 0.004$)
Edmiston, et al[37] 2015	100	Mean skin surface chlorhexidine concentrations in participants receiving electronic alerts following 1, 2, 3, 4, and 5 applications were 1,040.5, 1,334.4, 1,278.2, 1,643.9, and 1,803.1 µg/mL, respectively, whereas concentrations in the no-electronic alert group were 913.8, 1,240.0, 1,249.8, 1,194.4, and 1,364.2 µg/mL, respectively ($P < 0.001$)
Rhee, et al[33] 2018	63	Immediately and 6 h after cleansing, chlorhexidine cloths yielded higher residual chlorhexidine concentrations (2,500 and 1,250 µg/mL, respectively) and significantly lower bacterial densities compared with non-antiseptic cloths or cotton washcloths ($P < 0.001$)
Makhni, et al[34] 2018	16	When chlorhexidine gluconate cloths were used, bacterial counts were noted to be decreased, but this finding was not statistically significant ($P = 0.059$)

Abbreviation: MRSA, methicillin-resistant *Staphylococcus aureus*.

Zywiel and colleagues evaluated the incidence of deep SSIs in knee arthroplasty patients who used six chlorhexidine-impregnated cloths the evening before surgery and the morning of surgery without rinsing (dual application).[38] A single institution's database was reviewed in this level of evidence II study. A total of 136 patients who completed this protocol were compared with 711 who underwent standard in-hospital preparation only. The investigators defined a deep SSI as either a deep incisional or joint space infection occurring within 1 year of the surgical procedure and with the infection appearing to be related to the surgical procedure (ie, defined as an absence of a focus of infection or precipitating event unrelated to the index arthroplasty). They found that patients who complied with the skin preparation protocol had a considerably lower incidence of SSIs compared with those who underwent in-hospital preparation only. The 136 patients who used the dual-application protocol had no

SSIs compared with 21 infections in the 711 patients (3%).

Johnson and colleagues evaluated the incidence of surgical infections in TKA patients at a single institution using a preadmission dual-application chlorhexidine cloth protocol compared with a cohort of patients undergoing standard in-hospital perioperative preparation only.[19] In a level of evidence II study, a total of 478 patients who underwent the protocol were compared with 1,735 patients who did not. They found that the incidence of SSIs was significantly lower at approximately 1 year follow-up in patients who used the full at-home advance 2% chlorhexidine gluconate protocol when compared with the comparison group (ie, 0.6 compared with 2.2%, $P = 0.021$).

Kapadia and colleagues in a level of evidence II study further investigated the incidence of surgical infections in TKA patients at a single institution using a preadmission chlorhexidine cloth dual-application protocol compared with a

Table 2 Results of total knee arthroplasty studies		
Report	Subjects	Results
Eiselt,[42] 2009	736	Lower incidence of infections following total joint arthroplasty after implementation of chlorhexidine cloth use compared with before (1.59 vs 3.19%)
Zywiel, et al[38] 2011	847	Patients who used chlorhexidine cloths had a 0% incidence of SSIs compared with 3% for those who underwent in-hospital preparation only
Hogenmiller,[44] 2011	341	Found zero SSIs in the 7-month time period following implementation of chlorhexidine cloth use
Kapadia, et al[9] 2013	per 1,000	Annual net savings of approximately $2.1 million with use of chlorhexidine cloths at their institution, and annual US health care savings of potentially $3.18 billion
Johnson, et al[19] 2013	2,213	Patients who used chlorhexidine cloths had a 0.6% incidence of SSIs compared with 2.2% for those who did not ($P = 0.021$)
Farber, et al[43] 2013	3,715	Incidence of SSIs was similar in patients receiving (1.0%, 18 of 1,891) and

(continued on next page)

Table 2 (continued)		
Report	Subjects	Results
		not receiving (1.3%, 24 of 1,824) chlorhexidine cloth, though only one cloth application
Kapadi, et al[40] 2015	4,751	A total of 1,035 patients were compliant with a chlorhexidine cloth disinfection protocol (22%) compared with 3,716 who were not (78%)
Kapadia, et al[39] 2016	3,717	Patients who used chlorhexidine cloths had a 0.03% incidence of periprosthetic infections compared with 1.9% for those who did not ($P = 0.002$)
Kapadia, et al[41] 2016	554	There were seven infections in the non-chlorhexidine group (2.9%) vs one in the chlorhexidine group (0.4%)
Worden, et al[45] 2017	N/A	Found a marked reduction in the SSI rate from 1.28% to 0.78%

Abbreviations: N/A, not available; SSIs, surgical site infections.

cohort of patients undergoing standard in-hospital perioperative preparation only.[39] In their study of 3717 total patients who underwent primary or revision TKA and either used chlorhexidine cloths before surgery (991 patients) or did not (2,726 patients), the use of the cloths was found to be associated with a significantly reduced relative risk (RR) of periprosthetic infection at approximately 1 year surveillance (0.03 compared with 1.9%, $P = 0.002$).

The same investigators also studied the annual health care cost savings of implementing a preoperative chlorhexidine cloth treatment protocol.[9] In a level of evidence II study, they determined the rates of SSIs following TKA and the cost per revision procedure by analyzing reports from the National Healthcare Safety Network and previously published reports. They concluded that the cost-benefit of using chlorhexidine cloths at their institution per 1,000 TKA patients was a net savings of approximately $2.1 million and this was extrapolated to be greater than $2 billion in annual health care savings for the United States (ie, two-thirds reduction of periprosthetic annual cost of $3.18 billion).

Kapadia and colleagues evaluated the compliance with a chlorhexidine cloth disinfection protocol at their institution.[40] They reviewed their institutional database (level of evidence II) and analyzed 2,458 patients who underwent primary or revision THA as well as 2,293 patients who underwent primary or revision TKA. Compliance was assessed by instructing patients to remove adhesive stickers from the cloth packages at the time of disinfection and to affix them to the instruction sheet presented on the day of surgery. Their results demonstrated that a total of 1,035 patients were compliant (22%) compared with 3,716 who were not (78%). The demographics of the two groups were not found to be greatly different. This low compliance demonstrates the need to overly emphasize to patients the need to use these cloths.

These same investigators conducted a prospective randomized study to better assess the effect of the chlorhexidine cloths.[41] In analyses of primary hips, primary knees, revision hips, and revision knees (level of evidence I) with 275 patients in the chlorhexidine group and 279 in the non-chlorhexidine group, they found that there were seven deep periprosthetic infections in the non-chlorhexidine group (2.9%) versus one in the chlorhexidine group (0.4%). Thus, their prospective randomized study demonstrated the advantage of using chlorhexidine cloths.

A level of evidence I study by Eiselt confirmed the effects of the chlorhexidine cloths.[42] The implementation of a protocol wherein chlorhexidine cloths were applied the evening before and the morning of the surgery was evaluated at a single institution with a total of 736 joint arthroplasty procedures analyzed. The investigator found a lower incidence after patients started to use chlorhexidine cloths compared with patients who did not (1.59 vs 3.19%). This represented a greater than 50% decrease in the rate of SSIs. The study further demonstrated that this trend continued through the year after implementation.

One study did not demonstrate a statistically significant effect of chlorhexidine cloths.[43] In a one-application study (level of evidence II) without mention of compliance, Farber and colleagues retrospectively compared the SSI rates between total joint arthroplasty patients who used chlorhexidine cloths to those who did not. They reviewed 3,715 patients (1,660 THAs and 2,055 TKAs) from their institution. They did not see a positive effect of using the chlorhexidine-impregnated cloths as part of a preoperative preventative measure for patients undergoing primary lower extremity total joint arthroplasty. The 1-year incidence of SSIs was similar in patients receiving (1.0%, 18 of 1,891) and not receiving (1.3%, 24 of 1,824) chlorhexidine cloths. However, this study only used a single chlorhexidine application, which differed from all of the other studies that used a dual application technique.

Hogenmiller presented an investigation of whether 2% chlorhexidine cloths used the night before and morning of surgery prevented total joint arthroplasty SSIs.[44] A total of 341 patients were analyzed in a level of evidence III single-institution study. They found no SSIs in the 7-month time period following implementation of chlorhexidine cloth use.

Worden and colleagues reported on whether the use of chlorhexidine cloths the day of surgery decreased SSIs in TKA or THA patients as well as spine surgery patients.[45] All patients who underwent TKA or THA as well as spine surgery from April 1 through October 31, 2016 in a 168-bed acute care community hospital were included (level of evidence III). They found a marked reduction in the SSI rate, from 1.28% to 0.78% for the 6-month observation period.

In summary, 10 studies analyzing chlorhexidine cloths and their relationship with knee arthroplasty (or combined lower extremity arthroplasty with hip) were evaluated (see Table 2). Seven of 8 outcome studies showed a decreasing incidence of SSIs with the use of the cloths. The one report that did not still had a lower infection rate for the chlorhexidine cloth group (1.0 vs 1.3%, not significant), but this may not have been an appropriate comparison to the other seven studies, because they only used a single application. The remaining two reports discussed the substantial economic impact of chlorhexidine cloths and the need to improve on patient compliance.

Hip Arthroplasty
In the following section, the authors review the outcomes from three level of evidence II reports

Table 3 Results of hip arthroplasty studies		
Report	**Subjects**	**Results**
Johnson, et al[46] 2010	954	No surgical site infections in the chlorhexidine cloth users, whereas there were 14 (1.6%) for those receiving only standard preoperative skin preparation
Kapadia, et al[18] 2013	2,458	Statistically significant lower incidence of infections occurred in patients who used chlorhexidine cloths (3 infections, 0.5%) compared with patients who did not (32 infections, 1.7%) at approximately 1 year follow-up ($P = 0.04$)
Brown, et al[48] 2014	3,517	Rate of infections fell from 1.17 (25 of 2,130) to 0.5% (7 of 1,387) ($P = 0.045$)
Kapadia, et al[47] 2016	3,844	Patients who did not have preoperative chlorhexidine gluconate disinfection were shown to have a significantly higher risk of infections vs those who received chlorhexidine (1.62 compared with 0.6%, $P = 0.0226$)

Abbreviation: THAs, total hip arthroplasties.

and a lower level study on THA. Other combined knee and hip studies were discussed above in the knee arthroplasty section.

Johnson and colleagues evaluated the effectiveness of chlorhexidine-impregnated cloths in decreasing the incidence of deep periprosthetic hip arthroplasty infections in a multi-surgeon single-institution study.[46] In a level of evidence II study, a total of 954 patients were analyzed with 157 performing applications of chlorhexidine cloths the night before and the morning of surgery and the remaining 897 receiving only the standard preoperative skin preparation. There were no SSIs in the chlorhexidine cloth users, whereas 14 (1.6%) had infections in the comparison group.

Kapadia and colleagues investigated the incidence of SSIs in THA patients who used a dual application of chlorhexidine-impregnated cloth compared with patients who did not.[18] A total of 557 patients who used the chlorhexidine cloths and 1901 patients who did not were studied through a review of their institution's database (level of evidence II). They found a statistically significant lower incidence of infections occurring in patients who used the chlorhexidine cloths (3 infections, 0.5% when compared with patients who did not (32 infections, 1.7%) ($P = .04$), thus, demonstrating the efficacy of the chlorhexidine-impregnated cloths.

The above investigators also performed a larger level of evidence II study to determine if preadmission dual application of chlorhexidine cloths decreased the risk of SSIs in patients undergoing THA. A total of 3844 THA patients who either used chlorhexidine cloths before surgery (998 patients) or only underwent standard perioperative disinfection (2,846 patients) were

studied. Patients who did not use the preoperative chlorhexidine disinfection protocol were shown to have a significantly higher risk of infections for 1 year after surgery (1.62 compared with 0.6%, $P = 0.0226$).[47]

Brown and colleagues evaluated the effects of preoperative chlorhexidine use at home.[48] A total of 3,517 THA patients from a single center were investigated (level of evidence III). They compared the infection rates after implementation of this protocol to the rate of infection in the preceding 34 months. Their results demonstrated that the rate of hip infections fell from 1.17 (25 of 2,130) to 0.5% (7 of 1,387) ($P = 0.045$). They also found that the rate of infections caused by *S aureus* decreased from 0.66% to 0.22% over the same time period.

In summary, three level of evidence II articles and a lower level study all showed the positive effect of chlorhexidine cloth use for the prevention of SSIs after THAs (Table 3). Note that four other studies reporting on positive results of cloths after combined hip and knee arthroplasties were discussed in the preceding section.

Further Summary of Hip and Knee Arthroplasty Reports

In total, there were nine knee and hip arthroplasty clinical outcome studies (two level of evidence I and seven level of evidence II) on the effects of preoperative chlorhexidine cloth use. The specifics of the demographics (Table 4) and infection rates (Table 5) are detailed below.

Meta-Analysis

The meta-analysis included eight studies (15,323 patients) and demonstrated overall significant reductions with the dual application use of

Table 4
Demographics

Study	Combined Number of Patients	Age in Years, Mean (Range)	Sex: M:F	Mean Body Mass Index (kg/m²) (Range)
Eiselt,[42] 2009	736	N/A	N/A	N/A
Johnson, et al[46] 2010	954	58 (26–89)	1:1	29 (15–60)
Zywiel, et al[38] 2011	847	63 (20–90)	1:2	34 (17–39)
Johnson, et al[19] 2013	2213	63 (18–90)	1:1	34 (15–74)
Kapadia, et al[18] 2013	2,458	57 (12–106)	2:3	34 (15–77)
Farber, et al[43] 2013	3,715	64	4:5	N/A
Kapadia, et al[39] 2016	3,717	62	2:3	34
Kapadia, et al[41] 2016	554	62 (41–104)	1:2	32 (19–41)
Kapadia, et al[47] 2016	3,844	59	9:11	30

Abbreviations: F, female; M, male; N/A, not available

chlorhexidine cloths (0.42 vs 1.98%, $P < 0.05$) (**Table 6**). In addition, a meta-analysis was performed on six studies (14,033 patients) analyzing the infection incidence stratified by patient risk (**Table 7**). It found that the dual application of chlorhexidine cloths significantly reduced the rate in low- (0.5 vs 1%), medium- (0.3 vs 2.1%), and high-(0.7 vs 4.6%) risk patients ($P < 0.05$).

Other Surgical Specialties

Chlorhexidine cloth use has been analyzed in five studies (two level of evidence I, two level of evidence II, and one lower level unpublished study) in other surgical fields, which will now be summarized.

Murray and colleagues tested whether the home application of a 2% chlorhexidine gluconate cloth before shoulder surgery would be more efficacious than a standard shower of soap and water at decreasing the preoperative cutaneous levels of pathogenic bacteria on the shoulder.[49] In a multi-surgeon single-institutional randomized, prospective study (level of evidence I), they evaluated 100 consecutive patients, equally assigned to use 2% chlorhexidine gluconate-impregnated cloths (treatment group) or to shower with soap and water before surgery (control group). Their outcomes of interest were overall positive culture rates and the positive culture rates for coagulase-negative *Staphylococcus* at a minimum of 2 months follow-up. They found that the treatment group had an overall positive culture rate of 66%, whereas it was 94% in the control group ($P = 0.0008$). The positive culture rate for coagulase-negative *Staphylococcus* was 30 versus 70% for the treatment and control cohorts, respectively ($P = 0.0001$).

Table 5
Infection prevention success of chlorhexidine cloths stratified by patient risk

Study	Combined Number of Patients	Overall Infection Incidence	Low Risk	Medium Risk	High Risk
Eiselt,[42] 2009	736	1.59 vs 3.19%	N/A	N/A	N/A
Johnson, et al[46] 2010	954	0 vs 1.6%	0 vs 1.6%	0 vs 2.7%	0 vs 7.3%
Zywiel, et al[38] 2011	847	0 vs 3%	0 vs 1.6%	0 vs 2.4%	0 vs 7.3%
Johnson, et al[19] 2013	2,213	0.6 vs 2.2%	0.9 vs 1.1%	0.5 vs 2.4%	0 vs 4%
Kapadia, et al[18] 2013	2,458	0.5 vs 1.7%	0.6 vs 0.8%	0 vs 1.7%	2.5 vs 5.6%
Farber, et al[43] 2013	3,715	1.0 vs 1.3%	N/A	N/A	N/A
Kapadia, et al[39] 2016	3,717	0.03 vs 1.9%	0.5 vs 1%	0.2 vs 2.1%	0 vs 3.5%
Kapadia, et al[41] 2016	554	0.4 vs 2.9%	N/A	N/A	N/A
Kapadia, et al[47] 2016	3,844	0.6 vs 1.62%	0.5 vs 0.9%	0.6 vs 1.8%	1 vs 4.1%

Abbreviation: N/A, not available.

Table 6
Meta-analysis of overall infection incidence

Study	Combined Number of Patients	Overall Infection Incidence
Eiselt,[42] 2009	736	1.59 vs 3.19%
Johnson, et al[46] 2010	954	0 vs 1.6%
Zywiel, et al[38] 2011	847	0 vs 3%
Johnson, et al[19] 2013	2,213	0.6 vs 2.2%
Kapadia, et al[18] 2013	2,458	0.5 vs 1.7%
Kapadia, et al[39] 2016	3,717	0.03 vs 1.9%
Kapadia, et al[41] 2016	554	0.4 vs 2.9%
Kapadia, et al[47] 2016	3844	0.6 vs 1.62%
Pooled effect	15,323	0.42 vs 1.98% ($P < 0.05$)

Graling and colleagues conducted a prospective cohort study on the effectiveness of preoperative chlorhexidine gluconate cloths at reducing SSIs.[50] They implemented a practice change to use 2% chlorhexidine cloths preoperatively on all patients older than 2 months of age who were admitted through the main operating room preoperative area during a 4-month period. These patients were compared with baseline patients undergoing general and vascular surgery found in the National Surgical Quality Improvement Program database maintained by their surgery department (level of evidence II). A total of 335 patients who received the chlorhexidine cloths were compared with 284 patients who did not receive chlorhexidine cloth application. They defined a deep surgical wound infection as occurring at the operative site within 30 days of surgery if no implant was left in place or within 1 year if an implant was left in place. The infections also had to seem to be related to the surgery and involve tissue or spaces at or beneath the fascial layer. Their results indicated a statistically significant overall reduction of infections in the group that received a 2% chlorhexidine cloth application before surgery (7 infections (2.1%) compared with 18 (6.3%) without chlorhexidine cloths, $P = 0.01$).

Bak and colleagues evaluated the rate of SSIs after their institution implemented chlorhexidine gluconate-impregnated cloths as a preoperative antiseptic preparation in elective vascular surgery.[51] They reviewed 250 patients who used the chlorhexidine cloths preoperatively and compared them with 252 control patients who received chlorhexidine showers preoperatively before the implementation (level of evidence II). They evaluated SSIs within 30 days of operation and found no difference in the overall rate (5.6 vs 5.6%, $P = 1.00$), but the chlorhexidine shower group trended toward deeper infections (4 deep incisional and 2 organ space vs 0 and 1, respectively). In addition, the shower group had

Table 7
Meta-analysis of infection incidence stratified by patient risk

Study	Combined Number of Patients	Low Risk	Medium Risk	High Risk
Johnson, et al[46] 2010	954	0 vs 1.6%	0 vs 2.7%	0 vs 7.3%
Zywiel, et al[38] 2011	847	0 vs 1.6%	0 vs 2.4%	0 vs 7.3%
Johnson, et al[19] 2013	2,213	0.9 vs 1.1%	0.5 vs 2.4%	0 vs 4%
Kapadia, et al[18] 2013	2,458	0.6 vs 0.8%	0 vs 1.7%	2.5 vs 5.6%
Kapadia, et al[39] 2016	3,717	0.5 vs 1%	0.2 vs 2.1%	0 vs 3.5%
Kapadia, et al[47] 2016	3,844	0.5 vs 0.9%	0.6 vs 1.8%	1 vs 4.1%
Pooled effect	14,033	0.5 vs 1% ($P < 0.05$)	0.3 vs 2.1% ($P < 0.05$)	0.7 vs 4.6% ($P < 0.05$)

Table 8
Results of other surgical specialty studies

Report	Subjects	Results
Baxter et al,[53] 2009	1,098 orthopedic cases	Significant reduction in the SSI rate from 3.05% to 1.04% (*P* = 0.015)
Murray et al,[49] 2011	100 shoulder surgeries	Group treated with 2% chlorhexidine gluconate-impregnated cloths had an overall positive culture rate of 66%, whereas it was 94% in the control group (*P* = 0.0008)
Graling et al,[50] 2013	619 general and vascular surgery cases	Reduction of infection in the group that received a 2% chlorhexidine cloth application before surgery (7 infections (2.1%) compared with 18 (6.3%), *P* = 0.01)
Bak et al,[51] 2017	502 vascular surgery cases	Chlorhexidine shower group trended toward deeper infections and had significantly more dirty or infected surgical wounds (21.4 vs 10%, *P* < 0.01), antibiotic errors, including their redosing and timing (*P* < 0.02), and frequent perioperative hypothermia (22.2 vs 10%, *P* < 0.01)
Stone et al,[52] 2020	1,309 cesarean deliveries	A total of 10 of 516 (1.9%) patients in the chlorhexidine group and 17 of 502 (3.4%) patients in the placebo group were diagnosed with SSIs at 6 wk after cesarean delivery (relative risk, 0.57; 95% confidence interval, 0.26–1.24)

Abbreviation: SSI, surgical site infection.

significantly more dirty or infected surgical wounds (21.4 vs 10%, *P* < 0.01), antibiotic errors, including redosing and timing (*P* < 0.02), and frequent perioperative hypothermia (22.2 vs 10%, *P* < 0.01), suggesting that the use of chlorhexidine cloths led to shallower and cleaner infections.

Stone and colleagues investigated whether preadmission application of chlorhexidine gluconate-impregnated cloths may decrease SSIs after cesarean delivery.[52] In a single-institution level of evidence I study, they randomized 662 patients to use chlorhexidine cloths and 647 to use a placebo the night before and after a shower in the morning of the scheduled cesarean delivery. They found no significant difference in

SSIs by 6 weeks between the two groups (2.6 in the chlorhexidine group compared with 3.7% in the placebo group, *P* = 0.24). However, they found that the absolute difference in the rate of SSIs between the chlorhexidine and the placebo groups was −1.14%. In addition, when adjusting for full adherence to the protocol and those who were available for assessment, 10 of 516 (1.9%) patients in the chlorhexidine group and 17 of 502 (3.4%) patients in the placebo group were diagnosed with SSIs at 6 weeks after cesarean delivery (RR, 0.57; 95% confidence interval (CI), 0.26–1.24). The low RR and wide range of the CIs suggested to the authors that greater compliance may lead to enough power to achieve clinical significance.

Baxter and colleagues, in a level of evidence III study, investigated the effect of implementing 2% chlorhexidine non-rinse cloths for the "night-before and morning-of" site-specific skin preparation on orthopedic SSIs.[53] They analyzed 1,098 cases performed at a single institution. Their data analyses revealed a significant reduction in the SSI rates per 100 surgeries from 3.05% to 1.04% ($P = 0.015$).

In summary, five studies in other surgical fields also reported on the efficacy of chlorhexidine cloths in decreasing SSIs (Table 8). A total of three of the studies reported significant reductions in infections with the use of the chlorhexidine cloths. The remaining two both showed improved outcomes and positively trending results regarding the cloth applications reducing SSIs. However, they did not achieve significance, possibly due to their low power.

DISCUSSION

One of the most devastating complications after primary lower extremity total joint arthroplasties is periprosthetic infections.[3–6] Unfortunately, despite substantial infection prevention efforts, their rate has been increasing.[2,10] Ready-to-use, no-rinse, 2% chlorhexidine-impregnated cloths have shown excellent results for infection prophylaxis. Thus, the authors endeavored to conduct a literature review of studies on chlorhexidine cloths relating to the relevant surgical basic science studies, knee and hip arthroplasties, and other surgical fields. Almost every study that had reasonable power (>90%) and used a dual application approach showed positive results and improvement. All other studies demonstrated decreases in SSI rates or severity. A further meta-analysis of relevant studies comparing the results of dual application chlorhexidine cloths on lower extremity joint arthroplasties (15,323 patients) demonstrated significant reduction in SSI incidence (0.42 vs 1.98%, $P < 0.05$). In addition, a meta-analysis analyzing the infection incidence stratified by patient risk (14,033 patients) found that the dual application of chlorhexidine cloths significantly reduced the rate in low- (0.5 vs 1%), medium- (0.3 vs 2.1%), and high-(0.7 vs 4.6%) risk patients ($P < 0.05$).

This comprehensive review of surgeries contained all literature on chlorhexidine cloth applications in TKAs. Some TKA data were combined with THA results, but nevertheless, these findings should provide guidance for the audience.

This study is not without limitations. Some reports were underpowered and there is still the need for more level of evidence I studies. In addition, compliance was not always reported and, as particularly noted in one study, can be a major problem.[40] If compliance were optimized, even better results may have been achieved. Further work in this area is warranted.

SUMMARY

Based on the reports included in this review, it seems that the use of chlorhexidine cloths is appropriate for prophylaxis in a wide variety of surgeries. In knee and hip arthroplasties, preoperative use of chlorhexidine cloths has demonstrated favorable clinical outcomes in the systematic reviews. In addition, a detailed meta-analysis showed favorable outcomes in all arthroplasty studies. Also, there were similar favorable outcomes in reducing SSIs found in other general surgical fields. Further investigation into those specialties as well as even more medical applications would be appropriate for future studies. In summary, chlorhexidine cloths have demonstrated a reduction in SSIs, and the authors believe that their dual application with use the night before and the morning of surgery should be the standard of care.

CLINICS CARE POINTS

- use of chlorhexidine cloths is appropriate for prophylaxis in a wide variety of surgeries, especially lower extremity arthroplasties.
- Dual application use the night before and the morning of surgery should be the standard of care.
- Further investigation into other specialties as well as even more medical applications would be appropriate for future studies.

DISCLOSURE

Dr M.A. Mont is a board or committee member for The Knee Society and The Hip Society, receives research support from National Institutes of Health and is on the editorial board for the Journal of Arthroplasty, Journal of Knee Surgery, Surgical Technology International, and Orthopedics. Dr M.A. Mont also receives company support from 3M, Centrexion, Ceras Health, Flexion Therapeutics, Johnson & Johnson, Kolon TissueGene, NXSCI, Pacira, Pfizer-Lily, Skye

Biologics, SOLVD Health, Smith & Nephew, Stryker, MirrorAR, Peerwell, US Medical Innovations, and RegenLab. All other authors have no conflict of interest to disclose.

REFERENCES

1. Pabinger C, Lothaller H, Geissler A. Utilization rates of knee-arthroplasty in OECD countries. Osteoarthr Cartil 2015;23:1664–73.
2. Kurtz S, Ong K, Lau E, et al. Projections of primary and revision hip and knee arthroplasty in the United States from 2005 to 2030. J Bone Jt Surg - Ser A 2007. https://doi.org/10.2106/JBJS.F.00222.
3. Banerjee S, Kapadia BH, Mont MA. Preoperative skin disinfection methodologies for reducing prosthetic joint infections. J Knee Surg 2014. https://doi.org/10.1055/s-0034-1371771.
4. Kapadia BH, Berg RA, Daley JA, et al. Periprosthetic joint infection. Lancet 2016. https://doi.org/10.1016/S0140-6736(14)61798-0.
5. Jakobsson J, Perlkvist A, Wann-Hansson C. Searching for Evidence Regarding Using Preoperative Disinfection Showers to Prevent Surgical Site Infections: A Systematic Review. Worldviews Evidence-based Nurs 2011. https://doi.org/10.1111/j.1741-6787.2010.00201.x.
6. Parvizi J, Pawasarat IM, Azzam KA, et al. Periprosthetic joint infection: The economic impact of methicillin-resistant infections. J Arthroplasty 2010. https://doi.org/10.1016/j.arth.2010.04.011.
7. Bozic KJ, Lau E, Kurtz S, et al. Patient-related risk factors for periprosthetic joint infection and postoperative mortality following total hip arthroplasty in medicare patients. J Bone Jt Surg - Ser A 2012. https://doi.org/10.2106/JBJS.K.00072.
8. Bozic KJ, Ong K, Lau E, et al. Estimating risk in medicare patients with THA: An electronic risk calculator for periprosthetic joint infection and mortality hip. Clin Orthop Relat Res 2013. https://doi.org/10.1007/s11999-012-2605-z.
9. Kapadia BH, Johnson AJ, Issa K, et al. Economic evaluation of chlorhexidine cloths on healthcare costs due to surgical site infections following total knee arthroplasty. J Arthroplasty 2013. https://doi.org/10.1016/j.arth.2013.02.026.
10. Kurtz SM, Lau E, Watson H, et al. Economic burden of periprosthetic joint infection in the united states. J Arthroplasty 2012. https://doi.org/10.1016/j.arth.2012.02.022.
11. Springer BD, Cahue S, Etkin CD, et al. Infection burden in total hip and knee arthroplasties: an international registry-based perspective. Arthroplast Today 2017. https://doi.org/10.1016/j.artd.2017.05.003.
12. Mangram AJ, Horan TC, Pearson ML, et al. Guideline for Prevention of Surgical Site Infection, 1999. Centers for Disease Control and Prevention (CDC) Hospital Infection Control Practices Advisory Committee. Am J Infect Control 1999. https://doi.org/10.1016/S0196-6553(99)70088-X.
13. Percival SL, Emanuel C, Cutting KF, et al. Microbiology of the skin and the role of biofilms in infection. Int Wound J 2012. https://doi.org/10.1111/j.1742-481X.2011.00836.x.
14. Altemeier WA, Culbertson WR, Hummel RP. Surgical considerations of endogenous infections–sources, types, and methods of control. Surg Clin North Am 1968. https://doi.org/10.1016/S0039-6109(16)38448-1.
15. Noble WC. The production of subcutaneous staphylococcal skin lesions in mice. Br J Exp Pathol 1965; 46(3):254–62.
16. Feldman G, Fertala A, Freeman T, et al. Recent Advances in the Basic Orthopedic Sciences: Osteoarthritis, Infection, Degenerative Disc Disease, Tendon Repair and Inherited Skeletal Diseases. Recent Adv Orthop 2014. https://doi.org/10.5005/jp.books.12346_17.
17. Edmiston CE, Seabrook GR, Johnson CP, et al. Comparative of a new and innovative 2% chlorhexidine gluconate-impregnated cloth with 4% chlorhexidine gluconate as topical antiseptic for preparation of the skin prior to surgery. Am J Infect Control 2007. https://doi.org/10.1016/j.ajic.2006.06.012.
18. Kapadia BH, Johnson AJ, Daley JA, et al. Pre-admission Cutaneous Chlorhexidine Preparation Reduces Surgical Site Infections In Total Hip Arthroplasty. J Arthroplasty 2013. https://doi.org/10.1016/j.arth.2012.07.015.
19. Johnson AJ, Kapadia BH, Daley JA, et al. Chlorhexidine reduces infections in knee arthroplasty. J Knee Surg 2013. https://doi.org/10.1055/s-0032-1329232.
20. Kuyyakanond T, Quesnel LB. The mechanism of action of chlorhexidine. FEMS Microbiol Lett 1992. https://doi.org/10.1016/0378-1097(92)90211-6.
21. Leikin Jerrold B, Paloucek Frank P. Chlorhexidine gluconate", poisoning and toxicology handbook. 4th edition. Boca Raton, FL: Informa; 2008. p. 183–4.
22. Darouiche RO, Wall MJ, Itani KMF, et al. Chlorhexidine–Alcohol versus Povidone–Iodine for Surgical-Site Antisepsis. N Engl J Med 2010. https://doi.org/10.1056/nejmoa0810988.
23. Byrne DJ, Napier A, Cuschieri A. The value of whole body disinfection in the prevention of postoperative wound infection in clean and potentially contaminated surgery. A prospective, randomised, double-blind, placebo-controlled clinical trial. Surg Res Commun 1992;12(1):43–52.
24. Earnshaw JJ, Berridge DC, Slack RCB, et al. Do preoperative chlorhexidine baths reduce the risk of

infection after vascular reconstruction? Eur J Vasc Surg 1989. https://doi.org/10.1016/S0950-821X(89)80068-4.

25. Hayek LJ, Emerson JM, Gardner AMN. A placebo-controlled trial of the effect of two preoperative baths or showers with chlorhexidine detergent on postoperative wound infection rates. J Hosp Infect 1987. https://doi.org/10.1016/0195-6701(87)90143-5.

26. Rotter ML, Larsen SO, Cooke EM, et al. A comparison of the effects of preoperative whole-body bathing with detergent alone and with detergent containing chlorhexidine gluconate on the frequency of wound infections after clean surgery. J Hosp Infect 1988. https://doi.org/10.1016/0195-6701(88)90083-7.

27. Veiga DF, Damasceno CAV, Veiga-Filho J, et al. Randomized Controlled Trial of the Effectiveness of Chlorhexidine Showers Before Elective Plastic Surgical Procedures. Infect Control Hosp Epidemiol 2009. https://doi.org/10.1086/592980.

28. Wihlborg O. The effect of washing with chlorhexidine soap on wound infection rate in general surgery. A controlled clinical study. Ann Chir Gynaecol 1987;76(5):263–5.

29. Dizer B, Hatipoglu S, Kaymakcioglu N, et al. The effect of nurse-performed preoperative skin preparation on postoperative surgical site infections in abdominal surgery. J Clin Nurs 2009. https://doi.org/10.1111/j.1365-2702.2009.02885.x.

30. RANDALL PE, GANGULI L, MARCUSON RW. Wound Infection Following Vasectomy. Br J Urol 1983. https://doi.org/10.1111/j.1464-410X.1983.tb03371.x.

31. Burns PB, Rohrich RJ, Chung KC. The levels of evidence and their role in evidence-based medicine. Plast Reconstr Surg 2011. https://doi.org/10.1097/PRS.0b013e318219c171.

32. Ryder M. Evaluation of Chlorhexidine Gluconate (CHG) Delivered to the Skin Following Standard Pre-Op Prepping Protocols of 4% CHG Solution Versus No-Rinse 2% CHG Cloth. Am J Infect Control 2007. https://doi.org/10.1016/j.ajic.2007.04.016.

33. Rhee Y, Palmer LJ, Okamoto K, et al. Differential Effects of Chlorhexidine Skin Cleansing Methods on Residual Chlorhexidine Skin Concentrations and Bacterial Recovery. Infect Control Hosp Epidemiol 2018. https://doi.org/10.1017/ice.2017.312.

34. Makhni MC, Jegede K, Lombardi J, et al. No Clear Benefit of Chlorhexidine Use at Home Before Surgical Preparation. J Am Acad Orthop Surg 2018. https://doi.org/10.5435/JAAOS-D-16-00866.

35. Edmiston CE, Krepel CJ, Seabrook GR, et al. Preoperative Shower Revisited: Can High Topical Antiseptic Levels Be Achieved on the Skin Surface Before Surgical Admission? J Am Coll Surg 2008. https://doi.org/10.1016/j.jamcollsurg.2007.12.054.

36. Whitman TJ, Schlett CD, Grandits GA, et al. Chlorhexidine Gluconate Reduces Transmission of Methicillin-Resistant Staphylococcus aureus USA300 among Marine Recruits. Infect Control Hosp Epidemiol 2012. https://doi.org/10.1086/666631.

37. Edmiston CE, Krepel CJ, Spencer MP, et al. Preadmission application of 2% chlorhexidine gluconate (CHG): Enhancing patient compliance while maximizing skin surface concentrations. Infect Control Hosp Epidemiol 2015. https://doi.org/10.1017/ice.2015.303.

38. Zywiel MG, Daley JA, Delanois RE, et al. Advance pre-operative chlorhexidine reduces the incidence of surgical site infections in knee arthroplasty. Int Orthop 2011. https://doi.org/10.1007/s00264-010-1078-5.

39. Kapadia BH, Zhou PL, Jauregui JJ, et al. Does Preadmission Cutaneous Chlorhexidine Preparation Reduce Surgical Site Infections After Total Knee Arthroplasty? Clin Orthop Relat Res 2016. https://doi.org/10.1007/s11999-016-4767-6.

40. Kapadia BH, Cherian JJ, Issa K, et al. Patient Compliance with Preoperative Disinfection Protocols for Lower Extremity Total Joint Arthroplasty. Surg Technol Int 2015;26:351–4.

41. Kapadia BH, Elmallah RK, Mont MA. A Randomized, Clinical Trial of Preadmission Chlorhexidine Skin Preparation for Lower Extremity Total Joint Arthroplasty. J Arthroplasty 2016. https://doi.org/10.1016/j.arth.2016.05.043.

42. Eiselt D. Presurgical skin preparation with a novel 2% chlorhexidine gluconate cloth reduces rates of surgical site infection in orthopaedic surgical patients. Orthop Nurs 2009. https://doi.org/10.1097/NOR.0b013e3181a469db.

43. Farber NJ, Chen AF, Bartsch SM, et al. No infection reduction using chlorhexidine wipes in total joint arthroplasty. Clin Orthop Relat Res 2013. https://doi.org/10.1007/s11999-013-2920-z.

44. Hogenmiller J.R., Hamilton J., Clayman T., et al., Preventing Orthopedic Total Joint Replacement Surgical Site Infections through a Comprehensive Best Practice Bundle/Checklist. Poster presented at: APIC National Conference; June 2011; Baltimore, MD.

45. Worden C, Pihl D. Decreasing Surgical Site Infections (SSIs) by implementing a Nurse Driven Preoperative Protocol in a high risk surgical population. Poster presented at: APIC National Conference; June 2017; Portland, OR.

46. Johnson AJ, Daley JA, Zywiel MG, et al. Preoperative chlorhexidine preparation and the incidence of surgical site infections after hip arthroplasty. J Arthroplasty 2010. https://doi.org/10.1016/j.arth.2010.04.012.

47. Kapadia BH, Jauregui JJ, Murray DP, et al. Does Preadmission Cutaneous Chlorhexidine Preparation Reduce Surgical Site Infections After Total

Hip Arthroplasty? Clin Orthop Relat Res 2016. https://doi.org/10.1007/s11999-016-4748-9.

48. Brown L, Shelly M, Greene L, Pettis AM, Romig S. The Effect of Universal Intranasal Povidone Iodine Antisepsis on Total Joint Replacement Surgical Infections. Poster presented at: APIC National Conference; June 2017; Anaheim, CA.

49. Murray MR, Saltzman MD, Gryzlo SM, et al. Efficacy of preoperative home use of 2% chlorhexidine gluconate cloth before shoulder surgery. J Shoulder Elbow Surg 2011. https://doi.org/10.1016/j.jse.2011.02.018.

50. Graling PR, Vasaly FW. Effectiveness of 2% CHG Cloth Bathing for Reducing Surgical Site Infections. AORN J 2013. https://doi.org/10.1016/j.aorn.2013.02.009.

51. Bak J, Le J, Takayama T, et al. Effect of 2% Chlorhexidine Gluconate-Impregnated Cloth on Surgical Site Infections in Vascular Surgery. Ann Vasc Surg 2017. https://doi.org/10.1016/j.avsg.2016.11.011.

52. Stone J, Bianco A, Monro J, et al. Study To Reduce Infection Prior to Elective Cesarean Deliveries (STRIPES): a randomized clinical trial of chlorhexidine. Am J Obstet Gynecol 2020;223(1):113.e1–11.

53. Baxter M, Ables E, Allison R, Boren V, Brown B, Davis B, et al. Quality Improvement Program Ensures Preoperative Adherence to CDC SSI Prevention Guidelines and Reduces Orthopedic SSIs 66%. Poster presented at: IHI 21st Annual National Forum on Quality Improvement in Health Care; December 2009; Orlando, FL.

The Use of Proximal Femur Replacement for the Management of Oncologic Lesions in the Proximal Femur

A Review

Devon Tobey, MD*, Clayton Wing, MD,
Tyler Calkins, MD, Robert K. Heck, MD

KEYWORDS

• Proximal femur • Bone tumor • Limb salvage • Endoprosthetic reconstruction • Complications

KEY POINTS

- For tumors in the proximal femur, proximal femoral replacement with an endoprosthesis is a frequently used reconstruction method, with cited benefits being immediate weight bearing, effective pain control, and wide availability of implants.
- The overall rate of reoperation after proximal femoral replacement is variable, ranging from 5.3% to 47%, and reconstructive failures are common due to complications of the construct as well as issues related to oncologic care.
- Failure is defined as need for implant revision, fracture, soft-tissue reconstruction for joint stability, implant removal, and amputation.
- Failures are categorized into 5 types: soft-tissue failure, aseptic loosening, structural failure, infection, and tumor progression. Most failures are attributed soft-tissue problems and infection (6.8% and 5%, respectively).
- Newer prosthetic designs, including modular systems, silver coatings, and dual mobility liners, as well as changes in surgical technique (capsular repair/augmentation) are being developed to improve rates of treatment failures.

INTRODUCTION

The proximal femur is a common location of primary malignant tumors and metastatic carcinomas. The treatment of these lesions has changed dramatically during the last several decades and varies based on the nature of the lesion (primary vs metastatic). For patients with a primary malignancy of bone, the goal is resection and a stable reconstruction in hopes that the patient is cured. Conversely, the goal for patients with metastatic disease is not necessarily to cure but more so alleviation of pain and maintenance of function. The advent of newer, more effective chemotherapeutic agents has led to improved prognosis and longer life expectancy. As long-term patient survival rates continue to improve, there has been a push for limb salvage and more durable constructs. The optimum method for reconstruction remains controversial but segmental endoprostheses have had an increasingly major role in limb salvage and reconstruction following tumor surgery. Proximal femoral replacement has become a commonly used reconstruction method for both primary malignancy and metastatic

Department of Orthopaedic Surgery, Campbell Clinic Orthopaedics, 1211 Union Avenue, Memphis, TN 38104, USA
* Corresponding author.
E-mail address: devon.tobey@gmail.com

disease. The benefits of this treatment include immediate weight bearing, effective pain control, and wide availability of implants.

This study is a review to summarize the current concepts regarding the management of oncologic lesions in the proximal femur with proximal femur endoprostheses.

IMPLANT SURVIVORSHIP

Given that many patients with osseous oncologic lesions may have decreased life expectancy, implant failures leading to component revision may not surface because it is often more of a mid-to-long–term problem, and the implant can be predicted to outlive the patient. Only 2 studies within the literature have predicted implant survivorship past 10 years of follow-up.[1,2] Trovarelli and colleagues reported 82% predicted implant survivorship at 12 years in 38 patients who received proximal femoral replacement for oncologic conditions.[2] Kabukcuoglu and colleagues reported 57% predicted implant survivorship free from revision at 20 years in a cohort of 54 patients who underwent proximal femoral replacement for malignant conditions.[1] Five-year survivorship is widely variable within the literature, with the worst prediction being 58% implant survival and the best being 100% at 5-year (see Table 2). When expanded out to 10-year follow-up, rates of implant survivorship range from 58% to 93.8%. Predicted implant survivorship within individual studies are described within Table 2.

The overall rate of reoperation following proximal femoral replacement is widely variable as well at 5.3% to 47% (see Table 2). Six studies within this review reported on the reoperation rate in a cohort of 100 or more patients, ranging from 6.1% to 16% at mean follow-up of 1.3 to 7 years.[3–8] The study with the longest follow-up (7 years) in these larger cohort studies was by Houdek and colleagues (204 patients).[7] They found that the most common indication for component revision was aseptic femoral component loosening (8 of 22, 36.4%), whereas the most common indication for reoperation without component revision was irreducible hip dislocation (8 of 11, 72.7%). Interestingly, 7 of the 22 (31.8%) revision surgeries in this study were for conversion of hemiarthroplasty to total hip arthroplasty due to continued pain.

COMPLICATIONS

The goal of reconstruction using proximal femoral megaprostheses is to provide the patient with a stable construct that allows for early weight-bearing and provide satisfactory outcomes with a short recovery period. Although endoprosthetic replacement has come into favor for the management of proximal femoral lesions, there are inherent complications to a megaprosthesis construct as well as issues related to the patients oncologic care, and reconstructive failures are common. Additionally, these patients are oftentimes debilitated from their cancer with underlying malnourishment and on adjunctive therapies such as chemotherapy that can all increase the rates of complications.

Henderson and colleagues described a failure mode classification system that has been widely adapted as a means to categorize the modes, frequency, and timing of failure of these implants. In this multicenter, retrospective review of patients treated with a proximal femur endoprosthesis for the management of a tumor, they found 5 primary modes of failure (Table 1).[9] Failure was described as those requiring revision of the implant, periprosthetic fracture requiring fixation, the need for soft-tissue construction to restore joint stability, implant removal without revision, and amputation. These failures were categorized into mechanical and nonmechanical types of failure.

When looking at the time to failure from implantation, there was a mean failure time of 47 months but the mode of failure varied over time. The shortest mean time to failure was usually attributed to soft-tissue failure and the longest mean time to failure was due to aseptic loosening. In their study, total failure occurrences in proximal femoral replacements were seen in 20% of their cases.

A detailed list of all included studies within this review with description of their follow-up, proportion of cement use, femoral implant survival, rates of the 5 types of complications, and total reoperation rate are found in Table 2.

Type 1: Soft-Tissue Failure

Historically, instability of the hip has been the most common mode of failure of a proximal femoral endoprosthesis after tumor resection. It typically occurs early after the procedure. Dislocation is a well-documented complication of proximal femur replacement with rates ranging from 4% to 42%.[9,14,27,29] In a large series, by Ahlmann and colleagues, it occurred at a mean of 4.7 months postoperatively.[14] Another study quotes a 6% risk of experiencing a dislocation within 3 months after surgery.[24]

Table 1
Proximal femoral replacement survivorship and complications (Henderson classification) for proximal femoral oncologic lesions

Reference	Patients	Follow-up (Years)	Cemented Femurs (%)	Femoral Implant Survival	Type 1 (%)	Type 2 (%)	Type 3 (%)	Type 4 (%)	Type 5 (%)	Reoperation Rate (%)
Morris et al,[10] 1995	31	5.3	0	100% (8 y)	3	0	0	3.2	6.5	9.7
Zehr et al,[11] 1996	17	NR	100	58% (10 y)	17	5.9	11.8	5.9	5.9	47
Unwin et al,[3] 1996	263	3.8	100	93.8% (10 y)	NR	3.4	1.9	2.6	4.6	6.1
Kabukcuoglu et al,[1] 1999	54	9	100	57% (20 y)	11.1	11.1	0	1.9	1.9	16.7
Donati et al,[12] 2001	25	12.3	0	NR	4	8	4	4.2	4	16
Ilyas et al,[13] 2002	15	6.7	0	NR	20	6.7	0	13.3	6.7	40
Ahlmann et al,[14] 2006	96	4.9	100	82% (5 y)	3.1	0	0	3.1	3.1	NR
Farid et al,[15] 2006	52	10	100	82% (10 y)	5.8	9.6	0	3.8	1.9	13.5
Menendez et al,[16] 2006	96	1.5	100	82% (10 y)	3.1	0	0	3.1	3.1	9.4
Gosheger et al,[17] 2006	41	3.8	32	79% (5 y)	7.3	NR	0	19.5	NR	NR
Orlic et al,[18] 2006	44	9	0	NR	9	0	NR	NR	NR	NR
Finstein et al,[19] 2007	62	5	100	62% (10 y)	4.8	11.3	4.8	4.8	7	19
Selek et al,[20] 2008	45	NR	Mixed	NR	2.3	4.4	0	4.4	NR	6.7
Chandrasekar et al,[4] 2008	100	1.3	100	83% (5 y)	3	0	0	6	4	9
Potter et al,[21] 2009	61	4.6	100	93% (5 y)	6.6	3.3	0	4.9	0	9.8
Henderson et al,[9] 2011	403	NR	NR	NR	5.2	2.7	1	3	4	NR
Harvey et al,[5] 2012	113	1.3	100	100% (5 y)	9	0	0	9	NR	12.4
Pala et al,[22] 2013	32	4.2	8.8	58% (5 y)	9.4	0	0	9.4	9.4	NR
Calabro et al,[6] 2016	109	2.5	50.5	74% (9 y)	3.9	0	1	5.8	2.9	9.7
Houdek et al,[7] 2016	204	7	100	NR	7	3.9	NR	8	8	16
Johnson et al,[23] 2019a	26	6	100	NR	7.7	0	0	15	3.8	31
Sørensen et al,[24] 2019	26	NR	100	NR	6	0	0	0	NR	15.4
Trovarelli et al,[2] 2019	38	1.9	71	82% (12 y)	10.5	2.6	0	2.6	2.6	18
Yilmaz et al,[25] 2019	41	5	57	NR	7.3	0	14.6	14.6	14.6	29

(continued on next page)

Table 1
(continued)

Reference	Patients	Follow-up (Years)	Cemented Femurs (%)	Femoral Implant Survival	Type 1 (%)	Type 2 (%)	Type 3 (%)	Type 4 (%)	Type 5 (%)	Reoperation Rate (%)
Bischel et al,[26] 2020	45	1.4	NR	80% (6 y)	13.3	0	0	2.2	NR	11.6
Nooh et al,[27] 2020	47	3.7	100	92% (5 y)	8.5	4.3	0	4.2	10.6	NR
Gusho et al,[28] 2021	19	0.7	NR	92% (5 y)	0	0	0	5	NR	5.3
Toepfer et al,[29] 2021	58	4.4	Mixed	85% (10 y)	27.6	3.7	7.4	7.7	0	26
Sofulu et al,[8] 2022	111	2	41.4	97% (5 y)	1.75	1.8	0	2.6	2.7	6.1
Zavras et al,[30] 2022	58	2.4	86	88% (10 y)	12	0	9.8	1.7	NR	10.3
Zhang et al,[31] 2022[a]	16	3.9	0	94% (7 y)	18.8	0	0	12.5	NR	12.5
Bernthal et al,[32] 2010	86	5.4	100	56% (20 y)	4.7	4.7	0	1.2	8.1	20.9

Not reported (NR); Follow-up reported in mean years from surgery.
[a] All procedures done for salvage of failed fixation of malignant pathologic fractures.

Table 2
Henderson classification system segmental endoprosthetic failure

Type of Failure	Mode of Failure	Description
Mechanical		
Type 1	Soft-tissue failure	Instability, tendon rupture, or aseptic wound dehiscence
Type 2	Aseptic loosening	Clinical and radiographic evidence of loosening
Type 3	Structural failure	Periprosthetic or prosthetic fracture or deficient osseous supporting structures
Nonmechanical		
Type 4	Infection	Infection about endoprosthesis necessitating removal of device
Type 5	Tumor progression	Recurrence or progression of tumor with contamination of endoprosthesis

Stability of the hip can be influenced by variables associated with the implant, surgical technique, and the patient and their associated pathologic condition. In surgery involving lesions of the proximal femur, this sometimes necessitates a larger soft tissue resection and loss of capsular support or abductor musculature for joint stability. Means to counteract these concerns with stability have been suggested to include capsular reinforcement with synthetic material or the use of constrained liners or a dual mobility cup. In a multicenter study by Henderson and colleagues, they found that direct capsular repair was not associated with a decreased rate of instability.[9] However, in their 70 patients that had synthetic augmentation of the abductors there were no failures due to instability suggesting a trend toward protection against instability but it did not reach significance. Sofulu and colleagues described the split trochanteric osteotomy technique to preserve the abductors was associated with lower Trendelenberg gait positivity in the long term compared with trochanter removal but often the tumor dictates excision margins and this cannot be preserved.[8]

The analysis by Henderson and colleagues did show that age older than 60 years, female gender, and a diagnosis of a primary bone tumor predicted instability and that a posterolateral approach and the use of hemiarthroplasty were protective against instability.[9] Ahlmann and colleagues additionally demonstrated that bipolar implants had greater survivorship than total hip endoprostheses.[14] Many studies cited a nearly

3-fold increased risk of instability with the use of total hip arthroplasty versus bipolar hemiarthroplasty replacement.[14,16,26] In cases of acetabular resurfacing, the use of dual mobility implants has shown promise of lower rates of dislocation.[29,33]

Different postoperative regimens have been suggested to minimize the risk of instability including protective weight bearing and immobilization or bracing. These should be considered on a case-specific basis. Elderly women should be counseled on an increased risk of instability and would likely benefit from enhanced postoperative precautions such as abduction bracing.

Soft-tissue failure also incorporates the complication of wound dehiscence. This complication can be expected at higher rates in patients that are undergoing neoadjuvant or preoperative chemotherapy and radiation. Chemotherapy has been shown to inhibit wound healing because most chemotherapeutic agents impede the inflammatory phase of wound healing and thus disrupt cellular migration to the wound and regeneration of the extracellular matrix.[34] Radiation inhibits wound healing by disrupting the remodeling sequence. Early effects of radiation cause repetitive inflammation, which leads to increased accumulation of extracellular matrix but then inhibits functions of matrix metalloproteinases that remodel the matrix.[35] McDonald and colleagues showed that patients who did not receive any chemotherapy had a significantly lower complication rate compared with both

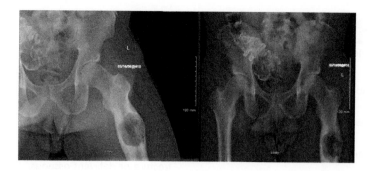

Fig. 1. Left proximal femur lesion. Biopsy confirmed a diagnosis of high-grade chondroblastic osteosarcoma.

adjuvant and neoadjuvant treatment, with the complication rate being highest in those treated with neoadjuvant therapy.[36] Thus, patients should be counseled on the incidence of these potential wound complications when considering proximal femoral replacements after tumor resection, particularly with the increased risk associated with adjuvant therapies.

Type 2: Aseptic Loosening

Durable fixation of the long-stemmed proximal femoral megaprosthesis to the diaphyseal femoral shaft can be a challenge due to high junctional forces at this interface. Rates of aseptic loosening of proximal femoral megaprostheses have ranged from 0% to 11.3% (see Table 2). Aseptic loosening was found to be the most common type of major complication in 3 of the 31 studies within this review. Earlier study has shown that it is more of a long-term complication, and patients with short-term follow up and lower survival rate may not be subjected to this type of failure.[3,31]

Improvements in cementing techniques and implant design have reduced the rate of loosening reported in contemporary literature,[7,23,24,27] compared with historical studies.[1,12,15,19] Cementless proximal femoral replacements have recently gained favor,[10,12,13,18,31] with some studies claiming this may decrease the risk of mid-to-late–term loosening due to bony ingrowth and osseointegration.[9,37]

Revisions for type 2 failures are challenging with a variety of suggested techniques. A recent study by Zhang and colleagues reported on 16 patients who underwent revision proximal femoral replacement (PFR) with cortical strut allograft and cementless fixation and had 94% predicted survivorship at 7 years postoperatively with no postoperative type 2 failures.[31] Another recent case report demonstrated good results with an extensive wire mesh, cerclage wiring, and impaction bone allograft with a cementless femoral PFR implant.[38] Other authors have suggested cemented femoral fixation techniques because the bone quality is likely to be especially poor in these cases.[23] Some have described cement in cement technique in cases in which the cement implant interface loosens. By keeping the cement mantle in place, conservation of native bone may be achieved which might otherwise be lost with removing cement before implanting a new revision PFR.

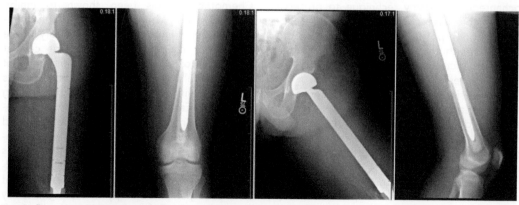

Fig. 2. Postoperative imaging of left proximal femoral replacement.

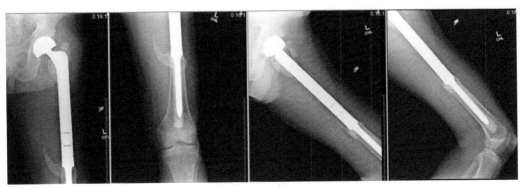

Fig. 3. Surveillance radiographs of left proximal femoral replacement.

Type 3: Structural Breakage

Similar to Type 2 failures in long stem proximal femoral megaprostheses, the high bending stresses at the prosthesis-to-bone and proximal body-to-stem interfaces in conjunction with potentially poor bone quality in oncologic patients can contribute to higher risk of periprosthetic or component fractures. Rates of these Type 3 failures were reported to range from 0% up to 14.6% at mean follow-up of 0.7 to 12.3 years in the studies included within this review (see Table 2).

Early designs of monoblock metal proximal femoral replacement implants that used cobalt-chrome proximal body and titanium stem distally had issues with stem fracture due to the difference in mechanical properties of the metal at a single stress riser junction.[39] Newer designs with improved implant cobalt-chrome and titanium interface manufacturing and some fully cobalt-chrome cemented designs as well as increased stem length and diameter have helped to decrease the risk of this implant fracture complication.[3,8,25,37] However, despite many titanium stems having similar modulus of elasticity to native diaphyseal shaft, periprosthetic femur fracture still remains a significant risk with some series reporting 8% to 15% rate.[11,25,29,30] To our knowledge, no studies have compared rates of these type of failures among cemented versus press-fit implants, and patients that can be appropriately indicated for cementless press-fit proximal femoral replacement may have inherently better bone quality.

Type 4: Infection

The most common major complication for proximal femoral replacement for malignancy is postoperative infection. The rate of infection varies across different studies with reported rates from 0% to 19.5% (see Table 2). Infection can result in significant financial and physical morbidity to the patient because it necessitates reoperation and often long-term antibiotic usage. In a retrospective study by Houdek and colleagues of 204 patients that underwent proximal femoral replacement, 8% of patients had infection in the postoperative period.[7] This was the most common complication seen in this case series. The reasoning behind the increased risk of infection is thought to be a combination of patient factors and the operation itself. Many oncology patients may be on chemotherapy, which can lead to an immunocompromised state

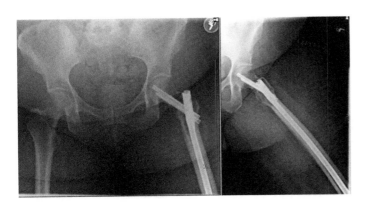

Fig. 4. Postoperative radiographs of prophylactic fixation of left proximal femur lesion with intramedullary nail.

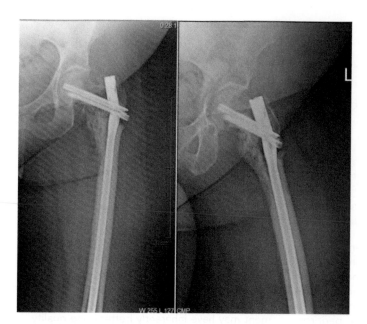

Fig. 5. Failure of intramedullary nail with progression of lesion.

and place them at a higher risk of infection. In addition, radiation treatment may predispose the surgical incision to wound breakdown and subsequent infection. Operative factors that increase the risk for infection include extensive surgical dissections, which result in longer exposure times of the incision and soft tissue defects that can create a dead space.[40] Even patients that have proximal femur replacement for non-neoplastic reasons seem to have increased infection rates. As shown in Table 2, most of the studies report a rate of infection that is higher than primary hip arthroplasty for osteoarthritis, which is around 2.5%.[41]

There have been efforts to decrease infection rates in these types of procedures, and one such area of research is the use of silver-coated prosthesis.[42,43] In a study of patients treated for sarcoma, Hardes and colleagues found that silver-coated megaprostheses had a significantly lower rate of infection compared with titanium implants.[43]

Type 5: Tumor Progression

There are times when failure of the proximal femoral replacement is related to local tumor progression. Earlier study has shown that this type of failure is more common if indicated for

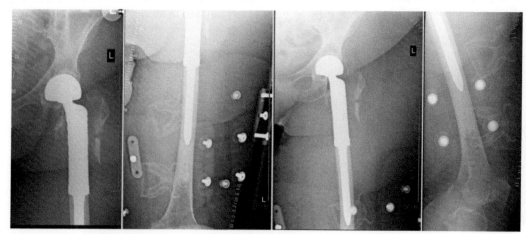

Fig. 6. Left proximal femoral replacement.

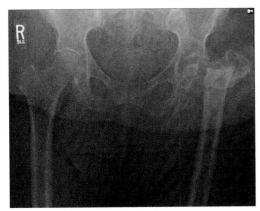

Fig. 7. Radiographs of left proximal femur pathologic fracture.

a primary tumor rather than resection related to metastatic disease within the proximal femur. It is thought that patients with metastatic disease may have higher rates of early mortality and the implant outlives patient survival.[9] Rates of failure for tumor progression are widely variable in the available literature ranging from 0% to 14.6% at 1.5 to 12.3 mean years of follow-up (see Table 2). The surgical treatment of this type of failure is typically amputation of the involved extremity rather than further revision procedures,[25] versus supportive adjuvant therapy for systemic disease.[27]

CASES

Here, we present a series of cases from our institution.

Case 1

RS is a 45-year-old gentleman who had a left proximal femur lesion and underwent needle biopsy, which confirmed a high-grade chondroblastic osteosarcoma (Fig. 1).

Workup for metastatic disease was negative, and the patient underwent 3 months of preoperative chemotherapy. He ultimately elected for wide resection and endoprosthetic reconstruction with hemiarthroplasty (Fig. 2) followed by postoperative chemotherapy.

The patient is now 14 years out from his reconstruction. He has had no recorded complications. He is ambulatory with a cane. He has had no recurrence of his osteosarcoma with regular PET and CT scans for surveillance. Fig. 3 depicts the patient's most recent imaging, which shows stable component position with heterotopic ossification at the proximal and distal aspects of the implant.

Case 2

SS presented as a 62-year-old woman with a painful lesion in her left proximal femur. She had known metastatic breast adenocarcinoma and underwent prophylactic fixation with intramedullary fixation (Fig. 4). She had appropriate radiation and medical treatment and did well for one and a half years postoperatively. She then began to experience left hip pain and was found to have a nondisplaced fracture at the anterior cortex of the proximal femur. This was followed for one and a half years without healing, and she was found to have progression of her metastatic lesion leading to severe pain and broken hardware (Fig. 5).

At this time, she underwent hardware removal, resection, and reconstruction with a proximal femoral replacement (Fig. 6). The hip capsule, obturator internus, and piriformis tendons were repaired. Postoperatively she wore an abduction brace for 6 weeks. At her last follow-up visit at 6 months postoperatively, she

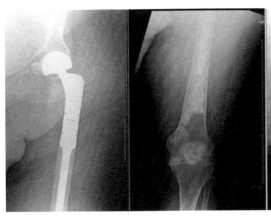
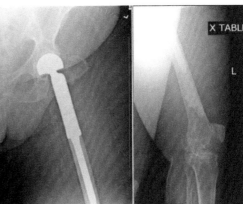

Fig. 8. Left femur proximal femoral replacement.

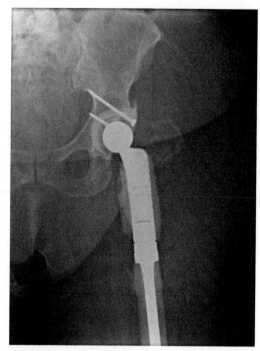

Fig. 9. Placement of antibiotic spacer for infected proximal femoral replacement.

proceed with proximal femoral replacement (Fig. 8). At her 2-week post-operative visit, her wound was healing appropriately and her staples were removed. She subsequently presented 10 days later with complaints of serous drainage from the wound. She underwent a debridement and irrigation with polyethylene exchange and placement of antibiotic beads into the wound. She was discharged from the hospital on 6 weeks of intravenous antibiotics. She subsequently did relatively well on suppressive oral antibiotic therapy until she sustained a fall at home around 7 months postoperatively and was closed reduced at an outside facility. She was placed into a hip abduction brace and continued physical therapy. She unfortunately sustained a second dislocation, and it was decided to revise her component with additional lengthening and anteversion of the component. She continued to have issues with draining sinuses and had recurrent dislocations and ultimately underwent a 2-stage revision with placement of an antibiotic spacer and conversion to a constrained liner component (Figs. 9 and 10).

She is now 8 months from her last revision and continues on her suppressive oral antibiotics and in physical therapy. She has not had any issues with wound drainage or instability. She will likely remain on lifelong suppressive antibiotic therapy due to her chronic infection and overall immunosuppressed state on systemic chemotherapy.

is doing well without any dislocations, signs of infection or significant pain.

Case 3

LE presented as a 73-year-old woman with a past medical history of metastatic breast cancer with long-standing left hip pain and inability to ambulate for the past few weeks. Radiographs at presentation demonstrated a left proximal femur pathologic fracture (Fig. 7).

Due to the chronicity of the fracture and previous radiation to the area, she elected to

SUMMARY

The proximal femur is a common location of primary malignant tumors and metastatic tumors. Treatment should attempt to provide local and systemic tumor control and requires multidisciplinary coordination. Goals of orthopedic

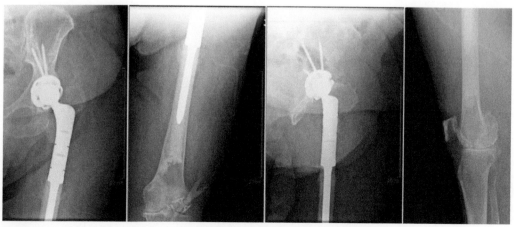

Fig. 10. Left proximal femoral replacement with constrained acetabular component.

management focus on tumor control, pain control, and ability to mobilize. The goals for management of these lesions are different for lesions of metastatic disease versus a primary malignancy of bone. Where the mainstay of treatment of primary malignancy is curative with resection and reconstruction, management of metastatic disease is not always to cure but instead to alleviate symptoms. Improvements in oncologic adjuvant therapies have led to better prognosis and longer life expectancy. As long-term patient survival for metastatic disease continues to improve, the use of megaprosthesis endoprosthetic reconstruction has continued to evolve in the treatment of proximal femoral oncologic lesions. Proximal femoral replacement has become an increasingly popular option for the reconstruction and management of proximal femoral lesions of both primary malignancy and metastatic disease. Although many studies cite acceptable results with proximal femoral replacement, there is still concern for reconstructive failure.

Classically, the Henderson classification system has been used to describe the mode of failure in segmental endoprostheses (Henderson and colleagues). In a review of the studies (see **Table 2**), most failures have been attributed to Type 1 (soft tissue) and Type 4 (infection) mechanisms. The cumulative rate of soft tissue failure and infection from these studies was 6.8% and 5%, respectively. Additionally, there is a trend toward higher rates of complication when megaprostheses are used for oncologic lesions of the proximal femur compared with nononcologic indications as well as in comparison to outcomes with primary total hip arthroplasty (Lindeque and colleagues). Host factors such as immunosuppression, radiation, and age are risk factors in this population that contribute to an increased risk of infection. Historically, there were much higher rates of Type 1 and Type 3 (structural) failures. Newer prosthesis designs including modular systems, silver coatings, and dual mobility liners, and changes in surgical technique (capsular repair/augmentation) have been implemented as means to counteract these failure modes.

This study aimed to consolidate the current research on the management of proximal femur oncologic lesions with endoprosthetic replacement. It is imperative that the treating orthopedic surgeon be aware of these failure modes and their impact on patient outcomes. Implant survivorship has been traditionally overshadowed by the fact that the implant typically outlived the patient. As patients are experiencing an improved prognosis and longer life expectancy, it has become even more important that the surgeon provide a durable construct. Additionally, one must account for host and surgical factors that could increase the risk for complication and should consider capsular repair or augmentation and supplemental bracing to minimize risk of dislocation in the immediate postoperative period.

CLINICS CARE POINTS

- Proximal femoral replacement is a common limb salvage reconstruction method for both primary and metastatic lesions of the proximal femur
- Benefits include immediate weight bearing, effective pain control and wide availability of implants
- There is a wide range of rate of reoperation, with 5 modes of failure classically described
- Newer developments in prosthesis design and surgical technique can help decrease the rate of treatment failures

DISCLOSURE

The authors have nothing to disclose.

REFERENCES

1. Kabukcuoglu Y, Grimer RJ, Tillman RM, et al. Endoprosthetic replacement for primary malignant tumors of the proximal femur. Clin Orthop Relat Res 1999;358:8–14.
2. Trovarelli GP, Cappallari A, Angelini A, et al. Proximal femoral reconstructions: A European "Italian" experience. A case series. Curr Orthop Pract 2019; 30(6):510–5.
3. Unwin PS, Cannon SR, Grimer RJ, et al. Aseptic loosening in cemented custom-made prosthetic replacements for bone tumours of the lower limb. J Bone Joint Surg Br 1996; 78(1):5–13.
4. Chandrasekar CR, Grimer RJ, Carter SR, et al. Modular endoprosthetic replacement for metastatic tumours of the proximal femur. J Orthop Surg Res 2008;3:50.
5. Harvey N, Ahlmann ER, Allison DC, et al. Endoprostheses last longer than intramedullary devices in proximal femur metastases. Clin Orthop Relat Res 2012;470(3):684–91.
6. Calabro T, Van Rooyen R, Piraino I, et al. Reconstruction of the proximal femur with a modular

resection prosthesis. Eur J Orthop Surg Traumatol 2016;26(4):415–21.

7. Houdek MT, Watts CD, Wyles CC, et al. Functional and oncologic outcome of cemented endoprosthesis for malignant proximal femoral tumors. J Surg Oncol 2016;114(4):501–6.

8. Sofulu O, Sirin E, Saglam F, et al. Implant survival and functional results of endoprosthetic reconstruction for proximal femoral metastases with pathological fractures. Hip Int 2022;32(2): 174–84.

9. Henderson ER, Groundland JS, Pala E, et al. Failure mode classification for tumor endoprostheses: retrospective review of five institutions and a literature review. J Bone Joint Surg Am 2011;93(5): 418–29.

10. Morris HG, Capanna R, Del Ben M, et al. Prosthetic reconstruction of the proximal femur after resection for bone tumors. J Arthroplasty 1995;10(3):293–9.

11. Zehr RJ, Enneking WF, Scarborough MT. Allograft-prosthesis composite versus megaprosthesis in proximal femoral reconstruction. Clin Orthop Relat Res 1996;(322):207–23.

12. Donati D, Zavatta M, Gozzi E, et al. Modular prosthetic replacement of the proximal femur after resection of a bone tumour a long-term follow-up. J Bone Joint Surg Br 2001;83(8):1156–60.

13. Ilyas I, Pant R, Kurar A, et al. Modular megaprosthesis for proximal femoral tumors. Int Orthop 2002; 26(3):170–3.

14. Ahlmann ER, Menendez LR, Kermani C, et al. Survivorship and clinical outcome of modular endoprosthetic reconstruction for neoplastic disease of the lower limb. J Bone Joint Surg Br 2006;88(6):790–5.

15. Farid Y, Lin PP, Lewis VO, et al. Endoprosthetic and allograft-prosthetic composite reconstruction of the proximal femur for bone neoplasms. Clin Orthop Relat Res 2006;442:223–9.

16. Menendez LR, Ahlmann ER, Kermani C, et al. Endoprosthetic reconstruction for neoplasms of the proximal femur. Clin Orthop Relat Res 2006;450: 46–51.

17. Gosheger G, Gebert C, Ahrens H, et al. Endoprosthetic reconstruction in 250 patients with sarcoma. Clin Orthop Relat Res 2006;450:164–71.

18. Orlic D, Smerdelj M, Kolundzic R, et al. Lower limb salvage surgery: modular endoprosthesis in bone tumour treatment. Int Orthop 2006;30(6): 458–64.

19. Finstein JL, King JJ, Fox EJ, et al. Bipolar proximal femoral replacement prostheses for musculoskeletal neoplasms. Clin Orthop Relat Res 2007;459: 66–75.

20. Selek H, Basarir K, Yildiz Y, et al. Cemented endoprosthetic replacement for metastatic bone disease in the proximal femur. J Arthroplasty 2008; 23(1):112–7.

21. Potter BK, Chow VE, Adams SC, et al. Endoprosthetic proximal femur replacement: metastatic versus primary tumors. Surg Oncol 2009;18(4): 343–9.

22. Pala E, Henderson ER, Calabro T, et al. Survival of current production tumor endoprostheses: complications, functional results, and a comparative statistical analysis. J Surg Oncol 2013; 108(6):403–8.

23. Johnson JD, Perry KI, Yuan BJ, et al. Outcomes of Endoprosthetic Replacement for Salvage of Failed Fixation of Malignant Pathologic Proximal Femur Fractures. J Arthroplasty 2019;34(4):700–3.

24. Sorensen MS, Horstmann PF, Hindso K, et al. Use of endoprostheses for proximal femur metastases results in a rapid rehabilitation and low risk of implant failure. A prospective population-based study. J Bone Oncol 2019;19:100264.

25. Yilmaz M, Sorensen MS, Saebye C, et al. Long-term results of the Global Modular Replacement System tumor prosthesis for reconstruction after limb-sparing bone resections in orthopedic oncologic conditions: Results from a national cohort. J Surg Oncol 2019;120(2):183–92.

26. Bischel OE, Suda AJ, Bohm PM, et al. En-Bloc Resection of Metastases of the Proximal Femur and Reconstruction by Modular Arthroplasty is Not Only Justified in Patients with a Curative Treatment Option-An Observational Study of a Consecutive Series of 45 Patients. J Clin Med 2020;9(3). https://doi.org/10.3390/jcm9030758.

27. Nooh A, Alaseem A, Epure LM, et al. Radiographic, Functional, and Oncologic Outcomes of Cemented Modular Proximal Femur Replacement Using the "French Paradox" Technique. J Arthroplasty 2020; 35(9):2567–72.

28. Gusho CA, Clayton B, Mehta N, et al. Internal fixation versus endoprosthetic replacement of the proximal femur for metastatic bone disease: Single institutional outcomes. J Orthop 2021;28:86–90.

29. Toepfer A, Strasser V, Ladurner A, et al. Different outcomes after proximal femoral replacement in oncologic and failed revision arthroplasty patients - a retrospective cohort study. BMC Musculoskelet Disord 2021;22(1):813.

30. Zavras AG, Fice MP, Dandu N, et al. Indication for Proximal Femoral Replacement Is Associated With Risk of Failure. J Arthroplasty 2022;37(5):917–24.

31. Zhang X, Tang X, Li Z, et al. Clinical and radiological outcomes of combined modular prothesis and cortical strut for revision proximal femur in giant cell tumor of bone patients. J Orthop Surg (Hong Kong) 2022;30(1). 10225536221095202.

32. Bernthal NM, Schwartz AJ, Oakes DA, et al. How long do endoprosthetic reconstructions for proximal femoral tumors last? Clin Orthop Relat Res 2010;468(11):2867–74.

33. Pennekamp PH, Wirtz DC, Durr HR. [Proximal and total femur replacement]. Oper Orthop Traumatol 2012;24(3):215–26.

34. Deptula M, Zielinski J, Wardowska A, et al. Wound healing complications in oncological patients: perspectives for cellular therapy. Postepy Dermatol Alergol 2019;36(2):139–46.

35. Haubner F, Ohmann E, Pohl F, et al. Wound healing after radiation therapy: review of the literature. Radiat Oncol 2012;7:162.

36. McDonald DJ, Capanna R, Gherlinzoni F, et al. Influence of chemotherapy on perioperative complications in limb salvage surgery for bone tumors. Cancer 1990;65(7):1509–16.

37. Lozano Calderon SA, Kuechle J, Raskin KA, et al. Lower Extremity Megaprostheses in Orthopaedic Oncology. J Am Acad Orthop Surg 2018;26(12): e249–57.

38. Schoof B, Jakobs O, Gehrke T, et al. Proximal femoral reconstruction after aseptic loosening following proximal femoral replacement for Ewing sarcoma: a case report with one-year follow-up. Hip Int 2014;24(1):103–7.

39. Dobbs HS, Scales JT, Wilson JN, et al. Endoprosthetic replacement of the proximal femur and acetabulum. A survival analysis. J Bone Joint Surg Br 1981;63-B(2):219–24.

40. Healey JH. CORR Insights: High infection rate outcomes in long-bone tumor surgery with endoprosthetic reconstruction in adults: a systematic review. Clin Orthop Relat Res 2013;471(6):2028–9.

41. Lindeque B, Hartman Z, Noshchenko A, et al. Infection after primary total hip arthroplasty. Orthopedics 2014;37(4):257–65.

42. Streitbuerger A, Henrichs MP, Hauschild G, et al. Silver-coated megaprostheses in the proximal femur in patients with sarcoma. Eur J Orthop Surg Traumatol 2019;29(1):79–85.

43. Hardes J, von Eiff C, Streitbuerger A, et al. Reduction of periprosthetic infection with silver-coated megaprostheses in patients with bone sarcoma. J Surg Oncol 2010;101(5):389–95.

Trauma

Heterotopic Ossification after Trauma

Jad Lawand, MS[a,1,*], Zachary Loeffelholz, MD[a,1], Bilal Khurshid, MS[b],
Eric Barcak, DO[a,1]

KEYWORDS

• Trauma • NSAIDs • Heterotopic ossification • Orthopedics • Hip arthroplasty
• Myositis ossificans

KEY POINTS

- Heterotopic ossification (HO) is most common after trauma, specifically traumatic brain injuries, spinal cord injuries, and thermal burns.
- HO may be treated prophylactically with nonsteroidal anti-inflammatory drugs and in some cases, radiation may be suitable.
- Recommendations regarding the timing of surgical intervention are variable, with some studies recommending against waiting for lesion maturation of the heterotopically ossified bone, whereas other studies support waiting for HO bone maturation before surgical intervention.
- Preoperative computed tomography scans can show entrapped Neurovascular structures as channels through the heterotopic bone that can be safely freed with Kerrison Rongeurs. First, identify normal anatomy and bone then resect from normal to abnormal to avoid injury to normal tissue.

INTRODUCTION

Heterotopic ossification (HO) refers to benign ectopic bone formation in soft tissue and is common following trauma surgery. Early symptom presentations include nonspecific findings such as erythema, swelling, loss of motion, occasional joint tenderness, and pain appearing 3 to 12 weeks post-trauma.[1] HO bone can restrict movement and progress into ankylosis that may necessitate surgical intervention. Forsberg and colleagues[2] reported an observed HO rate of 64.5% with extremity trauma necessitating orthopedic intervention in combat wounded patients. Most of the patients reported in the study are males under the age of thirty with high impact trauma involving blast injuries and gunshot wounds. No effective treatments for HO have been identified to date as the underlying cellular and molecular mechanisms have not been completely elucidated.[3] The current

literature suggests that the pathogenesis of HO involves inductive signaling pathways in inducible osteoprogenitor cells, yet attempts to locate systemic and local factors have not been successful.[3] Recent studies have uncovered the involvement of inflammatory signals and both the innate and adaptive immune system involvement in HO bone formation in response to soft-tissue damage.[4] The development of HO is likely complex and multifactorial. Although HO is not exclusive to trauma and orthopedic surgery, this article will discuss the current literature on the pathophysiology, prophylaxis, epidemiology, and treatment of postoperative HO following orthopedic trauma.

PATHOPHYSIOLOGY

Most of the studies on the pathophysiology of HO used animal models with the heredity version of HO, known as Fibrodysplasia

[a] Department of Orthopaedic Surgery, John Peter Smith Health Network, Fort Worth, Texas, USA; [b] Texas College of Osteopathic Medicine, Fort Worth, Texas, USA
[1]Present address: 1500 S Main St 2nd Floor, Fort Worth, TX 76104, USA.
* Corresponding author.
E-mail address: jadjlawand@gmail.com

Orthop Clin N Am 54 (2023) 37–46
https://doi.org/10.1016/j.ocl.2022.08.007
0030-5898/23/© 2022 Elsevier Inc. All rights reserved.

Ossificans Progressiva (FOP) providing mechanistic insights. Soft tissue prone to HO has an altered response to inflammation and injury-mediated cytokines. Mesenchymal stem cells are thought to be the major cell population involved in the formation of HO.[5] Beta morphogenic protein (BMP) and transforming growth factor-β are two cellular components responsible for regulating bone development through SMADs. In particular, BMP4 is of interest in HO as it is expressed in both bone and soft tissue. The levels of BMP4 are expressed in similar amounts in soft tissue and bones before fracture. However, following a femoral fracture in a rat model BMP4 expression increased tenfold in 6 h in soft tissue and BMP4 expression was unaffected in bone before returning to baseline in 72 h.[6] Moreover, BMP2 receptors are also of interest as their overexpression has been reported to induce HO.[7] However, eradicating BMP2 fails to prevent HO but it does delay onset.[8] Other nonspecific osteogenic progenitors including the expression of an angiogenic receptor Tie-2 have been shown to contribute to half of bone-forming cells with HO lesions.[8] These cells respond by differentiating through endochondral ossification and respond to BMP signaling.[9] Lin and colleagues[10] reported that the formation of HO appears to show intracellular homeostatic dependence by using Metformin to down-regulate AMP-activated protein kinase (AMPKA) inhibiting BMP and preventing trauma-induced HO in mice. Another study used pyrase locally at a burn site to prevent HO through the same mechanism by decreasing phosphorylated SMAD 1/5/8 in mesenchymal cells in vitro.[11] Moreover, nuclear retinoic acid receptor-g (RAR-g) agonists are also significant in the pathophysiology of HO due to their role in chondrogenesis.[12] Local micro-environment factors such as ischemic time, oxygen saturation, and mechanical stimulation also impact HO formation.[13,14] Therefore, the pathophysiology for HO induced following trauma surgery is likely multifactorial, with complex signaling pathways.

RISK FACTORS

Risk factors such as a prior history of HO, hypertrophic osteoarthritis, ankylosing spondylitis, and male gender have been linked to the development of HO in both THA and Open Reduction/Internal Fixation (ORIF) patients,[15] but many of these factors have also shown no increased HO in other studies. Risk factors that were more consistently found to increase HO prevalence were traumatic brain injury (TBI)

and prolonged mechanical ventilation. Patients requiring prolonged mechanical ventilation have an increased risk of developing HO with an odds ratio of 7.[16] One study showed an odds ratio of 8.6 for the development of HO following a TBI.[17] Following a TBI HO commonly affects the hip the most followed by the elbow, and rarely the knee. In contrast, the order of HO following an Spinal cord injury (SCI) more commonly affects the hip, knee, and elbow below the site of injury respectively. Hip flexors and abductors are more commonly affected than extensors or adductors.[18] Different surgical approaches have different rates of postoperative HO development. A meta-analysis comparing anterior and posterior surgical approaches to Pipkin I and II fractures of the femoral head reported a statistically significant 22% risk increase in the postoperative frequency of HO formation with the posterior approach compared with the anterior approach.[19] For acetabular fractures, the surgical approach has been implicated in the incidence of HO with the iliofemoral approach having the greatest risk of HO, followed by the Kocher–Langenbeck approach, and the ilioinguinal approach with the lowest risk of HO.[20–23] Interestingly, in patients with polytrauma with an associated head injury, HO occurred adjacent to the initial fracture zone. Whereas, in cases of polytrauma without an associated head injury, HO occurred in regions without any signs of injury.[24]

LAB FINDINGS

In early stages of HO, serum alkaline phosphatase level is elevated (3.5 × normal) but returns to physiologic levels in later stages of maturation.[25] It is important to note that age-adjusted levels of serum alkaline phosphatase do not increase in children during any stage of HO bone formation. Therefore, serum findings for the purpose of HO are only useful in ruling out bone mineralization disorders. A urinary increase of Prostaglandin E2 (PGE2) levels 24 h following trauma can be suggestive of HO. prophylaxis should be considered for those patients (Fig. 1).[26]

IMAGING

A distinguishing feature of trauma-induced HO bone formation is the appearance of an ectopic bone fragment with a peripheral ossification site. It is important to differentiate early stages of HO from conditions for which it is commonly

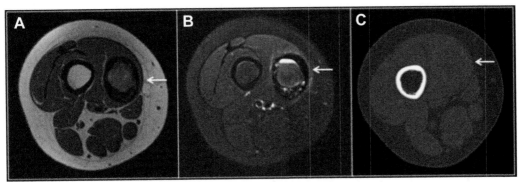

Fig. 1. Axial T1 (*A*), STIR (*B*), and CT (*C*) showing myositis ossificans (*arrow*) in the vastus medialis. (*From* Saad A, Azzopardi C, Patel A, Davies AM, Botchu R. Myositis ossificans revisited - The largest reported case series. J Clin Orthop Trauma. 2021 Mar 13;17:123-127. https://doi.org/10.1016/j.jcot.2021.03.005. PMID: 33816108; PMCID: PMC7995649.)

misdiagnosed including osteosarcoma and osteomyelitis.[27,28] Osteosarcomas have a central ossification site detected on imaging and are commonly seen in the metaphysis of long bones and don't typically occur following trauma.[29] During the early stages of bone mineralization, HO is indistinguishable from dystrophic calcification (DC) in imaging. As the mineralization process progresses, DC will remain as a nonossified amorphous calcification with a hazy ill-defined appearance that increases in density over time, whereas HO will develop into laminar bone.[28,30] Radiography and CT scans remain the most commonly used imaging modality for staging HO due to their cost-effectiveness and practicality. However, they are only sensitive to HO 6 weeks post-traumatic incident.[28] MRI can be used to confidently diagnose HO bone during the maturation stage only, presenting as a cancellous fat bone hyperintense of T1- and T2-weighted images with a hypointense rim of cortical bone.[31] Triple phase bone scans are the most sensitive imaging modality providing detections as early as 2.5 weeks following traumatic events through an increase in vascularity and radioactivity on potential HO sites.[32] To distinguish HO from osteomyelitis on bone scintigraphy ^{67}Ga uptake in HO is proportional to the uptake of 99mTc-diphosphonates, in contrast to the relatively greater ^{67}Ga uptake characteristic of osteomyelitis.[33] Ultrasonography (US) allows for bedside examination of soft tissues providing a convenient imaging modality for the detection of HO as a hyperechoic mass with an acoustic shadow and irregular muscular surrounding.[34] Furthermore, US grayscale values were shown to indicate a further progression of HO bone maturity.[34]

HIP

There are several events that can precipitate HO of the hip: thermal burns, hip arthroplasty, neurologic injury, and spinal cord injuries.[5] The reported occurrence of HO due to hip arthroplasty occurs in approximately 40% of patients after surgery.[5] The hip is the most common site of HO after a spinal cord injury, with the knee, elbow, and shoulder following.[5] Most of the HO does not necessitate clinical intervention, but severe HO can lead to decreased range of motion of the hip and pain.[35] The formation of HO is divided into classes using the Brooker classification system (I–IV). Class I of HO is small pieces of ossified bone floating within the soft tissue of the hip. Class II of HO is described as the bone spurs originating from the bone with at least 1 cm between bone surfaces. In the case of the hip, this will either be the pelvis or the proximal femur. Class III of HO consists of larger bone spurs that leave less than 1 cm between bony surfaces and Class IV of HO shows complete ankylosing and fusion between the bony surfaces.

There are several risk factors associated with HO of the hip: gender, prior occurrence, and osteoarthritis. Males are twice as likely as females to present with HO, however, women with osteoarthrosis show the same prevalence of HO as their male counterparts. Furthermore, any individual that has had an HO once before is far more likely to present with one later (Fig. 2).[36]

KNEE

Postoperative HO can arise from surgical trauma with the treatment of floating knee injuries.

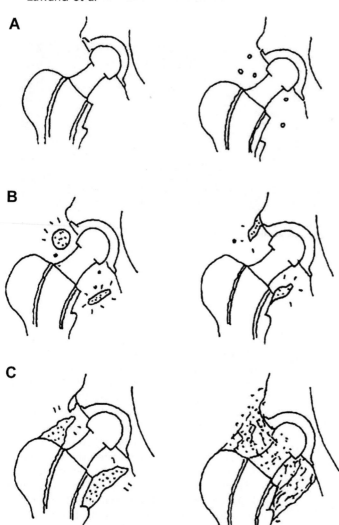

Fig. 2. (A) Normal (left); Class 1 of HO: islands of bone start to form within the soft tissue (right). (B) Advancement of Class 1 of HO consists of larger islands of bone (left); Grade 2 of HO consists of bone spur formation with a gap of greater than 1 cm between pelvis and femur (right). (C) Grade 3 shows the continued growth of bone spurs, now with less than 1 cm gap between pelvis and femur (left); Grade 4 shows ankylosis of the hip joint (right). From Della Valle AG, Ruzo PS, Pavone V, Tolo E, Mintz DN, Salvati EA. Heterotopic ossification after total hip arthroplasty: a critical analysis of the Brooker classification and proposal of a simplified rating system. J Arthroplasty. 2002;17(7):870-875.

Floating knee injuries are a flail knee joint that is due to fracturing of the shafts or metaphysis of the femur and tibia. These kinds of fractures are typically caused by a high impact or high-velocity injury and are typically treated with antegrade tibial intramedullary nailing/ipsilateral antegrade or retrograde femoral intramedullary nailing. Between these two treatment modalities, there was a significantly higher development and severity of HO in the retrograde group versus the antegrade group (90% vs 43%).[37] Despite the higher rates of HO formation and severity in the retrograde group, the study concluded that this increased severity is unlikely to affect range of motion.

SHOULDER

Clinically significant HO in the shoulder is rare but can cause severe impairment in daily activities.

Fuller and colleagues[38] retrospectively reviewed HO bone excision in 11 shoulders following a TBI. Significant improvements were seen in the Range of Motion (ROM) in all three planes, the HO bone occurred most frequently in motion interfaces, ligaments, and joint capsules, and HO recurrence was reported in 3/11 shoulders. Prophylactic use of nonsteroidal anti-inflammatory drugs (NSAIDs) for primary shoulder arthroplasty did not reduce postoperative HO, it is only indicated in patients with cuff tear arthropathy.[39] In patients with early HO in the shoulder post-SCI, a single-dose radiation 7 Gy and 6–15 MV therapy was used as an alternative treatment, resulting in no HO recurrence or adverse side effects reported during the follow-up period.[40] Male sex and dislocation as the initial injury all increase the risk of HO formation, whereas surgical treatment method, patient age, and fracture pattern were unpredictive.[41]

ELBOW

Direct trauma is the most frequent cause of HO in the elbow, and the incidence is positively correlated with the magnitude of injury.[42] The prevalence of postoperative trauma-induced HO on the proximal radius and ulna is 37%, and 42% on the distal humerus.[43,44] Other causes that can contribute to the development of HO in the elbow include thermal burns and injuries that precipitate general HO development risk below the level of injury (TBI, and spinal cord injury). HO is the most common cause of elbow contracture.[45] Despite variations in different populations, the overall incidence of HO postoperatively in the elbow is 28.7% in the adult population.[46] Floating elbow injuries accounted for the largest prevalence of HO, followed by combined olecranon and radial head fractures.[47] The collateral ligaments are the most common site of HO in the elbow.[47] Elbow ankylosis secondary to HO although rare causes significant disability in flexion and extension in HO bone anterior and posterior to the humeroulnar joint, respectively. Surgical open release of complete ankylosis secondary to HO has shown a significant arc improvement from 0° to 113.4° on average and mean pronation and supination improved from 34° to 52° and 51° to 76° respectively.[48] The excision of HO bone secondary to thermal injury also resulted in a significant improvement in ROM with an average gain of 80° from 0° in flexion and extension.[49] Despite minor variation in ROM improvements in different etiologies, surgical excision of HO bone in the elbow is effective.[50] The average complication rate of HO bone resection in the elbow is 22.6% with an 11.6% HO recurrence, ulnar nerve injury, and infection[50] Patients with brain injury had the most complications (27.5%), and burn patients had the fewest (16.4%).[50] Although HO, in general, does disproportionately affect men, the sex difference is less pronounced in the elbow joint.[47] Risk factors for clinically relevant HO include dislocation and surgery delay.[47] The use of any form of prophylaxis decreased the incidence of HO bone formation in comparison to the group without any prophylaxis with an odds ratio of 0.51, $P < .001$.[46] Therefore, prophylaxis should be considered in high-risk populations.

PEDIATRICS

The incidence of trauma-induced HO in the pediatric population following a TBI is 3% - 20% without variation between sex.[51,52] Clinically significant HO in children develops in 4 months on average.[51] Traumatic events that have been attributed to HO bone formation in children include near drowning, strangulation, cerebral hemorrhage, hydrocephalus, and spinal cord injury.[51] Serum alkaline phosphatase levels do not increase beyond age-normalized values in children under less than 20 during HO maturation.[51] Prophylaxis should be considered for children in a persistent vegetative state (PVS) as approximately 12% of all children in a PVS for 30 days or more developed HO bone.[51] Neurogenic HO rates are lower in children with an incidence rate of 8% compared with 20% in the adult population respectively.[53,54] To the best of our knowledge, no studies have identified an optimal time to excise the HO bone in children. Kluger and colleagues[51] suggested waiting for a minimum of 1 year before excision. Risk factors for HO following trauma surgery in children and adolescents include being older than 11 years and comatose for over 7 days, children with two or more extremity fractures, and spasticity.[52] In children, HO bone forms in the hip and knee most frequently, followed by shoulder, elbow, and nonjoint sites.[52] Following burns HO bone commonly forms on the elbow directly affected by the burn.[55] Gaur and colleagues[55] reported their management of HO bone excision following burn trauma in children. Surgical excision of HO bone in the elbow was done when the arc of motion was less than 50%. HO bone formed in a subset of patients with burns directly on the joint affected by the burn, no HO recurrence was reported during the follow-up period. Interestingly, the authors used pain resolution reported by surgical candidates to gauge HO bone maturity as the basis of excision timing.[55] Surgical recommendations include abandoning the use of a single posterior midline incision on the elbow through burned skin in favor of a multi-incision approach. The postoperative findings support the use of alternating splints to increase the arc of motion as opposed to the series of continuous passive motion. Furthermore, the position of elbow immobilization should be considered as it may impact the location of the HO bone. They reported a 0.25% prevalence of clinically significant HO bone causing a severe restriction ROM in burned children while studies reported an incidence of 0.1% to 3.3% but did not separate statistics from the pediatric population.[55,56] Radiation prophylaxis is not deemed suitable for the pediatric population due to the risks inherent with radiation on premature bone.

PROPHYLAXIS

NSAIDs can be used for HO prophylaxis in individuals at risk if no contraindications are present. Selective COX-2 inhibitors can also be used in place of nonselective NSAIDs if gastrointestinal disturbances are reported. Selective and nonselective NSAIDs are equally effective in prophylaxis.[57,58] Indomethacin has been tested with varying outcomes. Some studies show a decrease in the incidence of HO with indomethacin prophylaxis,[59,60] whereas others show no difference in HO incidence with indomethacin prophylaxis following THA.[61,62] In a prospective randomized trial, Brooker grade III to IV ossification occurred in nine of 59 patients (15.2%) in the Indomethacin group and 12 of 62 (19.4%) in the placebo group 3 months following the stabilization of their acetabular fractures through the posterior Kocher-Langenbeck approach[63] Those studies show no statistical significance between the groups. Indomethacin is commonly prescribed at a dose of 75 mg twice a day or 25 mg three times a day for 10 days to 6 weeks postoperatively.[5]

Other medications that have been used for HO prophylaxis include bisphosphonates with the use of etidronate in particular. Although one meta-analysis pointed to the efficacy of bisphosphonates in halting the progression of HO when administered before HO bone appears radiographically,[64] another meta-analysis reported no significant difference with the use of bisphosphonates on the incidence of HO although the effect size in that study was noted to be inconclusive.[63] More prospective studies need to be done on the use of bisphosphonates for HO prophylaxis following SCI, and TBI. Etidronate can be initiated orally, as intravenous administration provided no additional protection for HO prophylaxis.[64] The literature does not support the use of bisphosphonates for the treatment of HO after it appears radiographically.

Some studies reported local radiation therapy and indomethacin provide equal effectiveness as prophylaxis in preventing HO formation following surgical treatment of acetabular fractures through a posterior or extensile approach.[65] A systematic review compared local radiation therapy with indomethacin prophylaxis performed an underpowered meta-analysis suggesting that radiation therapy is superior to indomethacin with an HO incidence of 3% to 8% in acetabular fractures respectively.[66] Radiation can be administered at a dose of 700 to 800 cGy within a 24-h preoperative to 72-h postoperative period with equal prophylactic potential.[65] However, to the extent of our knowledge, no study has looked at the use of radiation therapy for HO in other joints.

Although radiation can be beneficial for HO prophylaxis, it remains controversial due to the cost, access, and possibility of increasing solid tumor risk. The most concerning potential side effect of radiation therapy for HO prophylaxis is carcinogenesis with no attributable cases documented to date. This may be due to the latency for radiation-induced tumors typically being greater than 10 years. It is possible that the lack of documented secondary malignancies is partially attributable to the relatively small number of patients who are followed up with long enough to develop them and the relatively low radiation dose used for HO prophylaxis.

For ORIF acetabular fractures, one study concluded that a revision of the surgical approach to include the debridement of the gluteus minimus necrotic muscle did not yield benefits in HO incidence, severity, and recurrence rate,[67] whereas another study stated debriding the necrotic gluteus minimus muscle did lower HO formation while treating acetabular fractures through a Kocher–Langenbeck approach.[68]

TREATMENT

If the patient experiences a significant joint mobility impairment, vascular or peripheral nerve entrapment caused by the HO bone, then surgical excision can be considered once the lesion is completely mature.[33] Indications for completely mature HO bone include the appearance of a bony cortex on a radiographic scan, sharp demarcations from surrounding tissue, decreased activity on a three-phase bone scan, formation of trabecular bone, and the normalization of C-reactive protein (CRP) and Alkaline phosphatase (ALP). The typical HO bone is considered mature 6 months after general trauma, 1 year after spinal cord injury, and 1.5 years after TBI.[69] However, the resection timeline following a TBI for HO bone is becoming controversial as some studies find no significant difference in HO recurrence following an early excision.[70–72] Classically, it has been accepted that HO should not be surgically resected until the bone formation is mature. In a systematic review, Chalidis and colleagues[70] compared early versus late surgical resection of HO in patients with TBI and showed no difference between the two groups in recurrence rates or overall gain of range of motion postoperatively. This study did not discreetly define the early or late time frame, but did recommend against watchful waiting for lesion maturation in the treatment of HO. A retrospective analysis reported a significant improvement in elbow functionality in patients that received HO excision early (<12 months) reflected by improvements in the Mayo Elbow Performance Score.[73]

The two surgical approaches for HO bone excision include the arthroscopic approach and the open approach.

Arthroscopy is suitable for when the HO bone is located peripherally and is easily accessible. This approach is minimally invasive with less blood loss, a lower risk of infection, and a faster recovery time. A radiofrequency ablation device and grasper are used to excise the HO bone while causing minimal damage to the surrounding tissue.[74] A burr can be used to divide the bone into smaller pieces that are more manageable with the arthroscopic approach. It is also important to note that the HO bone can be vascularized and bleed during resection. This approach can also address any concurrent intra-articular pathologies including femoroacetabular impingement syndrome or Labral Tears.[74]

Open approaches are more commonly used for the treatment of HO. Open approaches are also recommended when arthroscopy cannot adequately treat the HO or the location is unsafe to treat through a scope, such as proximity to a neurovascular structure. A preoperative computed tomography (CT) scan with three-dimensional reconstructions can be helpful for operative planning as well as identifying any surrounding structures that may be entrapped by the HO.[75] If there is a neurovascular structure encased in the heterotopic bone, often a channel can be seen running through HO on the CT. In this instance, a Kerrison Rongeur can be helpful in debriding the heterotopic bone and freeing the neurovascular structure without injury. The open approach can many times use the same incision as the index procedure, but it should be extensile enough to expose the whole HO lesion and allow for identification/protection of any neurovascular structures and normal anatomy. The HO can be excised en bloc or it can be excised in a piecemeal fashion through a smaller approach with the use of rongeurs and osteotomes. Identifying normal anatomy/bone and then working from normal to abnormal can prevent accidental injury to native tissue. After excision of the HO, a bleeding bed of healthy tissue remains and meticulous hemostasis is recommended. Intraoperative fluoroscopy can be used as well to aid in identifying

HO and the completeness of resection. Scar tissue excision and manipulation may be warranted during the procedure to address any contractures. In general, secondary prophylaxis with radiation and or NSAIDs is recommended to decrease the recurrence of HO after surgical excision.

To the best of our knowledge, the only study that compared the different outcomes of arthroscopic, open, and combined approaches for the excision of ectopic bone is a retrospective review of HO excision in the elbow.[76] The use of either indomethacin or radiation therapy for HO prophylaxis was reported in 84% of individuals in the open group, 92% of individuals in the combined group, and 95% in the arthroscopic group. No significant difference in postoperative complications was noted with the three approaches. However, the arthroscopic approach had the highest rate of HO recurrence or worsening contracture.[76] The study also highlights the importance of switching to multiple incisions medial and lateral as opposed to a single posterior incision with the open approach to minimize raising skin flaps, and the creation of a small posteromedial skin incision for ulnar nerve decompression prophylaxis.[76,77] Altogether, the study reported a decrease in the rate of major complications and reoperation with the open approach from 35% and 34% respectively to approximately 10% from 1997 to 2005 through the preventative measures described.[76]

Contraindications to the arthroscopic HO bone excision include:

1. Bony ankylosis.[76]
2. Radioulnar stenosis.[76]
3. Ossification greater than 50% of the collateral ligament.[76]
4. Extensive hardware.[76]
5. HO bone located near a major nerve comprising a safe excision via arthroscopic excision on CT.[78]

SUMMARY

Many factors have been implicated in predisposing to HO, but the main factors that have consistently been validated are the need for prolonged mechanical ventilation and TBI. There needs to be more research done on the efficacy of NSAIDs and radiation therapy as prophylactic agents because there are conflicting results in the literature, but many studies do advocate for their efficacy and safety and may be used in patients who are at higher risk of HO. Surgical excision of HO through an open, arthroscopic, or combined approach are all viable options for the treatment of HO but the timing of excision remains debated. In regard to future direction in HO research, the pathophysiology and mechanisms underlying HO are still being elucidated as are the novel therapeutic agents that could potentially target and alter these pathways through pharmacologic intervention.[7,8]

DISCLOSURE

The authors of this article have nothing to disclose.

REFERENCES

1. Cipriano CA, Pill SG, Keenan MA. Heterotopic ossification following traumatic brain injury and spinal cord injury. J Am Acad Orthop Surg 2009;17(11):689–97.
2. Forsberg JA, Pepek JM, Wagner S, et al. Heterotopic ossification in high-energy wartime extremity injuries: prevalence and risk factors. J Bone Joint Surg Am 2009;91(5):1084–91.
3. Xu R, Hu J, Zhou X, et al. Heterotopic ossification: Mechanistic insights and clinical challenges. Bone 2018;109:134–42.
4. Kraft CT, Agarwal S, Ranganathan K, et al. Trauma-induced heterotopic bone formation and the role of the immune system: A review. J Trauma Acute Care Surg 2016;80(1):156–65.
5. Ranganathan K, Loder S, Agarwal S, et al. Heterotopic Ossification: Basic-Science Principles and Clinical Correlates. J Bone Joint Surg Am 2015;97(13):1101–11 [published correction appears in J Bone Joint Surg Am. 2015 Sep 2;97(17):e59. Wong, Victor C [corrected to Wong, Victor W]].
6. Yaoita H, Orimo H, Shirai Y, et al. Expression of bone morphogenetic proteins and rat distal-less homolog genes following rat femoral fracture. J Bone Miner Metab 2000;18(2):63–70.
7. Krishnan L, Priddy LB, Esancy C, et al. Delivery vehicle effects on bone regeneration and heterotopic ossification induced by high dose BMP-2. Acta Biomater 2017;49:101–12.
8. Prados B, Del Toro R, MacGrogan D, et al. Heterotopic ossification in mice overexpressing Bmp2 in Tie2+ lineages. Cell Death Dis 2021;12(8):729.
9. Lounev VY, Ramachandran R, Wosczyna MN, et al. Identification of progenitor cells that contribute to heterotopic skeletogenesis. J Bone Joint Surg Am 2009;91(3):652–63.
10. Lin H, Shi F, Jiang S, et al. Metformin attenuates trauma-induced heterotopic ossification via inhibition of Bone Morphogenetic Protein signalling. J Cell Mol Med 2020;24(24):14491–501.
11. Peterson JR, De La Rosa S, Eboda O, et al. Treatment of heterotopic ossification through remote ATP hydrolysis. Sci Transl Med 2014;6(255):255ra132.
12. Shimono K, Tung WE, Macolino C, et al. Potent inhibition of heterotopic ossification by nuclear retinoic acid receptor-γ agonists. Nat Med 2011;17(4):454–60 [published correction appears in Nat Med. 2012 Oct;18(10):1592].
13. Hung SP, Ho JH, Shih YR, et al. Hypoxia promotes proliferation and osteogenic differentiation potentials of human mesenchymal stem cells. J Orthop Res 2012;30(2):260–6.
14. Kusuma GD, Carthew J, Lim R, et al. Effect of the Microenvironment on Mesenchymal Stem Cell Paracrine Signaling: Opportunities to Engineer the Therapeutic Effect. Stem Cells Dev 2017;26(9):617–31.
15. Corrigan CM, Greenberg SE, Sathiyakumar V, et al. Heterotopic ossification after hemiarthroplasty of the hip - A comparison of three common approaches. J Clin Orthop Trauma 2015;6(1):1–5.
16. Firoozabadi R, O'Mara TJ, Swenson A, et al. Risk factors for the development of heterotopic ossification after acetabular fracture fixation. Clin Orthop Relat Res 2014;472(11):3383–8.
17. Baschera D, Rad H, Collopy D, et al. Incidence and clinical relevance of heterotopic ossification after internal fixation of acetabular fractures: retrospective cohort and case control study. J Orthop Surg Res 2015;10:60.
18. Mavrogenis AF, Soucacos PN, Papagelopoulos PJ. Heterotopic ossification revisited. Orthopedics 2011;34(3):177. https://doi.org/10.3928/01477447-20110124-08.
19. Wang CG, Li YM, Zhang HF, et al. Anterior approach versus posterior approach for Pipkin I and II femoral head fractures: A systemic review and meta-analysis. Int J Surg 2016;27:176–81.
20. Firoozabadi R, Alton T, Sagi HC. Heterotopic Ossification in Acetabular Fracture Surgery. J Am Acad Orthop Surg 2017;25(2):117–24.
21. Johnson EE, Kay RM, Dorey FJ. Heterotopic ossification prophylaxis following operative treatment of acetabular fracture. Clin Orthop Relat Res 1994;305:88–95.
22. Alonso JE, Davila R, Bradley E. Extended iliofemoral versus triradiate approaches in management of associated acetabular fractures. Clin Orthop Relat Res 1994;305:81–7.
23. Bray TJ, Esser M, Fulkerson L. Osteotomy of the trochanter in open reduction and internal fixation of acetabular fractures. J Bone Joint Surg Am 1987;69(5):711–7.
24. Pape HC, Lehmann U, van Griensven M, et al. Heterotopic ossifications in patients after severe blunt trauma with and without head trauma: incidence

and patterns of distribution. J Orthop Trauma 2001; 15(4):229–37.

25. Orzel JA, Rudd TG. Heterotopic bone formation: clinical, laboratory, and imaging correlation. J Nucl Med 1985;26(2):125–32.

26. Schurch B, Capaul M, Vallotton MB, et al. Prostaglandin E2 measurements: their value in the early diagnosis of heterotopic ossification in spinal cord injury patients. Arch Phys Med Rehabil 1997;78(7):687–91.

27. Siegel MJ. Magnetic resonance imaging of musculoskeletal soft tissue masses. Radiol Clin North Am 2001;39(4):701–20.

28. Mujtaba B, Taher A, Fiala MJ, et al. Heterotopic ossification: radiological and pathological review. Radiol Oncol 2019;53(3):275–84.

29. Ritter J, Bielack SS. Osteosarcoma Ann Oncol 2010; 21(Suppl 7). vii320-vii325.

30. Hwang ZA, Suh KJ, Chen D, et al. Imaging Features of Soft-Tissue Calcifications and Related Diseases: A Systematic Approach. Korean J Radiol 2018; 19(6):1147–60.

31. Zagarella A, Impellizzeri E, Maiolino R, et al. Pelvic heterotopic ossification: when CT comes to the aid of MR imaging. Insights Imaging 2013;4(5):595–603.

32. Svircev JN, Wallbom AS. False-negative triple-phase bone scans in spinal cord injury to detect clinically suspect heterotopic ossification: a case series. J Spinal Cord Med 2008;31(2):194–6.

33. Shehab D, Elgazzar AH, Collier BD. Heterotopic ossification. J Nucl Med 2002;43(3):346–53.

34. Wang Q, Zhang P, Li P, et al. Ultrasonography Monitoring of Trauma-Induced Heterotopic Ossification: Guidance for Rehabilitation Procedures. Front Neurol 2018;9:771.

35. Hug KT, Alton TB, Gee AO. Classifications in brief: Brooker classification of heterotopic ossification after total hip arthroplasty. Clin Orthop Relat Res 2015;473(6):2154–7.

36. Iorio R, Healy WL. Heterotopic ossification after hip and knee arthroplasty: risk factors, prevention, and treatment. J Am Acad Orthop Surg 2002;10(6):409–16.

37. Kent WT, Shelton TJ, Eastman J. Heterotopic ossification around the knee after tibial nailing and ipsilateral antegrade and retrograde femoral nailing in the treatment of floating knee injuries. Int Orthop 2018;42(6):1379–85.

38. Fuller DA, Mani US, Keenan MA. Heterotopic ossification of the shoulder in patients with traumatic brain injury. J Shoulder Elbow Surg 2013;22(1):52–6.

39. Boehm TD, Wallace WA, Neumann L. Heterotopic ossification after primary shoulder arthroplasty. J Shoulder Elbow Surg 2005;14(1):6–10.

40. Sautter-Bihl ML, Hültenschmidt B, Liebermeister E, et al. Fractionated and single-dose radiotherapy for heterotopic bone formation in patients with spinal cord injury. A phase-I/II study. Strahlenther Onkol 2001;177(4):200–5.

41. Cirino CM, Chan JJ, Patterson DC, et al. Risk factors for heterotopic ossification in operatively treated proximal humeral fractures. Bone Joint J 2020;102-B(4):539–44.

42. Hastings H 2nd, Graham TJ. The classification and treatment of heterotopic ossification about the elbow and forearm. Hand Clin 1994;10(3):417–37.

43. Foruria AM, Augustin S, Morrey BF, et al. Heterotopic ossification after surgery for fractures and fracture-dislocations involving the proximal aspect of the radius or ulna. J Bone Joint Surg Am 2013; 95(10):e66.

44. Foruria AM, Lawrence TM, Augustin S, et al. Heterotopic ossification after surgery for distal humeral fractures. Bone Joint J 2014;96-B(12):1681–7.

45. Salazar D, Golz A, Israel H, et al. Heterotopic ossification of the elbow treated with surgical resection: risk factors, bony ankylosis, and complications. Clin Orthop Relat Res 2014;472(7): 2269–75.

46. Herman ZJ, Edelman DG, Ilyas AM. Heterotopic Ossification After Elbow Fractures. Orthopedics 2021;44(1):10–6.

47. Hong CC, Nashi N, Hey HW, et al. Clinically relevant heterotopic ossification after elbow fracture surgery: a risk factors study. Orthop Traumatol Surg Res 2015;101(2):209–13.

48. Chen S, Liu J, Cai J, et al. Results and outcome predictors after open release of complete ankylosis of the elbow caused by heterotopic ossification. Int Orthop 2017;41(8):1627–32.

49. Tsionos I, Leclercq C, Rochet JM. Heterotopic ossification of the elbow in patients with burns. Results after early excision. J Bone Joint Surg Br 2004;86(3): 396–403.

50. Lee EK, Namdari S, Hosalkar HS, et al. Clinical results of the excision of heterotopic bone around the elbow: a systematic review. J Shoulder Elbow Surg 2013;22(5):716–22.

51. Kluger G, Kochs A, Holthausen H. Heterotopic ossification in childhood and adolescence. J Child Neurol 2000;15(6):406–13.

52. Hurvitz EA, Mandac BR, Davidoff G, et al. Risk factors for heterotopic ossification in children and adolescents with severe traumatic brain injury. Arch Phys Med Rehabil 1992;73(5):459–62.

53. Mital MA, Garber JE, Stinson JT. Ectopic bone formation in children and adolescents with head injuries: its management. J Pediatr Orthop 1987; 7(1):83–90.

54. Sullivan MP, Torres SJ, Mehta S, et al. Heterotopic ossification after central nervous system trauma: A current review. Bone Joint Res 2013;2(3):51–7.

55. Gaur A, Sinclair M, Caruso E, et al. Heterotopic ossification around the elbow following burns in children: results after excision. J Bone Joint Surg Am 2003;85(8):1538–43.

56. Crawford CM, Varghese G, Mani MM, et al. Hetero-topic ossification: are range of motion exercises contraindicated? J Burn Care Rehabil 1986;7(4): 323–7.

57. Xue D, Zheng Q, Li H, et al. Selective COX-2 inhib-itor versus nonselective COX-1 and COX-2 inhibitor in the prevention of heterotopic ossification after total hip arthroplasty: a meta-analysis of rando-mised trials. Int Orthop 2011;35(1):3–8.

58. Zhu XT, Chen L, Lin JH. Selective COX-2 inhibitor versus non-selective COX-2 inhibitor for the pre-vention of heterotopic ossification after total hip arthroplasty: A meta-analysis. Medicine (Baltimore) 2018;97(31):e11649.

59. Joice M, Vasileiadis GI, Amanatullah DF. Non-ste-roidal anti-inflammatory drugs for heterotopic ossi-fication prophylaxis after total hip arthroplasty: a systematic review and meta-analysis. Bone Joint J 2018;100-B(7):915–22.

60. Kjaersgaard-Andersen P, Schmidt SA. Total hip arthroplasty. The role of antiinflammatory medica-tions in the prevention of heterotopic ossification. Clin Orthop Relat Res 1991;263:78–86.

61. Griffin SM, Sims SH, Karunakar MA, et al. Hetero-topic ossification rates after acetabular fracture sur-gery are unchanged without indomethacin prophylaxis. Clin Orthop Relat Res 2013;471(9): 2776–82.

62. Karunakar MA, Sen A, Bosse MJ, et al. Indometacin as prophylaxis for heterotopic ossification after the operative treatment of fractures of the acetabulum. J Bone Joint Surg Br 2006;88(12):1613–7.

63. Yolcu YU, Wahood W, Goyal A, et al. Pharmaco-logic prophylaxis for heterotopic ossification following spinal cord injury: A systematic review and meta-analysi. Clin Neurol Neurosurg 2020; 193:105737.

64. Aubut JA, Mehta S, Cullen N, et al, ERABI Group; Scire Research Team. A comparison of heterotopic ossification treatment within the traumatic brain and spinal cord injured population: An evidence based systematic review. NeuroRehabilitation 2011;28(2):151–60.

65. Archdeacon MT, d'Heurle A, Nemeth N, et al. Is preoperative radiation therapy as effective as post-operative radiation therapy for heterotopic ossifica-tion prevention in acetabular fractures? Clin Orthop Relat Res 2014;472(11):3389–94.

66. Blokhuis TJ, Frölke JP. Is radiation superior to indo-methacin to prevent heterotopic ossification in acetabular fractures?: a systematic review. Clin Orthop Relat Res 2009;467(2):526–30.

67. Chen MJ, Tigchelaar SS, Wadhwa H, et al. Gluteus Minimus Debridement During Acetabular Fracture Surgery Does Not Prevent Heterotopic Ossification-A Comparative Study. J Orthop Trauma 2021;35(10):523–8.

68. Rath EM, Russell GV Jr, Washington WJ, et al. Gluteus minimus necrotic muscle debridement di-minishes heterotopic ossification after acetabular fracture fixation. Injury 2002;33(9):751–6.

69. Garland DE. A clinical perspective on common forms of acquired heterotopic ossification. Clin Orthop Relat Res 1991;263:13–29.

70. Chalidis B, Stengel D, Giannoudis PV. Early exci-sion and late excision of heterotopic ossification af-ter traumatic brain injury are equivalent: a systematic review of the literature. J Neurotrauma 2007;24(11):1675–86.

71. Beingessner DM, Patterson SD, King GJ. Early exci-sion of heterotopic bone in the forearm. J Hand Surg Am 2000;25(3):483–8.

72. McAuliffe JA, Wolfson AH. Early excision of hetero-topic ossification about the elbow followed by radi-ation therapy. J Bone Joint Surg Am 1997;79(5): 749–55.

73. He SK, Yi M, Zhong G, et al. Appropriate excision time of heterotopic ossification in elbow caused by trauma. Acta Orthop Traumatol Turc 2018; 52(1):27–31.

74. Turner EHG, Goodspeed DC, Spiker AM. Excision of Heterotopic Ossification around the Hip: Arthro-scopic and Open Techniques. Arthrosc Tech 2021; 10(4):e1179–86.

75. Nauth A, Giles E, Potter BK, et al. Heterotopic ossi-fication in orthopaedic trauma. J Orthop Trauma 2012;26(12):684–8.

76. Bachman DR, Fitzsimmons JS, O'Driscoll SW. Safety of Arthroscopic Versus Open or Combined Heterotopic Ossification Removal Around the Elbow. Arthroscopy 2020;36(2):422–30.

77. Blonna D, Wolf JM, Fitzsimmons JS, et al. Prevention of nerve injury during arthroscopic capsulectomy of the elbow utilizing a safety-driven strategy. J Bone Joint Surg Am 2013;95(15):1373–81.

78. Bachman DR, Kamaci S, Thaveepunsan S, et al. Pre-operative nerve imaging using computed tomogra-phy in patients with heterotopic ossification of the elbow. J Shoulder Elbow Surg 2015;24(7):1149–55.

Fixation Principles for Pathologic Fractures in Metasatic Disease

Kendall M. Masada, MD[a],*, Sarah R. Blumenthal, MD[a],
Cara A. Cipriano, MD, MSc[b]

KEYWORDS

- Fixation • Pathologic • Fractures • Bone tumors • Metastases

KEY POINTS

- Primary malignant bone tumors must be ruled out before operative intervention for pathologic fracture.
- Pathologic bone has impaired healing and requires additional fixation strategies.
- Adjuvant therapies are critical in the management of pathologic fractures.

INTRODUCTION

Pathologic fractures occur in response to altered bone physiology, resulting in compromised mechanical properties owing to an underlying lesion. The root cause can be either benign or malignant, primary (ie, bone sarcoma) or secondary (ie, metastatic disease). These entities require different treatments, and the consequences of a missed diagnosis can be devastating; therefore, proper evaluation of the lesion is essential before surgery. The broad differential diagnosis includes metastases, benign bone tumors and tumor-like conditions (eg, fibrous dysplasia, aneurysmal bone cyst, giant cell tumor), bone sarcomas (eg, osteosarcoma, Ewing's sarcoma, secondary sarcoma), and lymphoproliferative diseases (eg, myeloma and lymphoma). Of these, metastasis is the leading cause of pathologic fracture and 500 times more common than primary bone sarcoma.[1] This article will, therefore, focus mainly on pathologic fractures secondary to metastatic disease; however, a diagnosis of primary bone sarcoma must be excluded before intervention.

An estimated 1.9 million people will be diagnosed with cancer in 2022. More than half of these diagnoses will involve cancers that metastasize to bone, the most common being breast, prostate, lung, renal, and thyroid carcinomas.[2] Overall, the skeleton is the third most common site of metastatic disease after the lungs and liver, and the most frequent sites for metastasis include the spine, pelvis, proximal femur and proximal humerus.[3,4] In the United States, the cumulative incidence of bone metastases after the date of diagnosis is 2.9% at 30 days, 4.8% at 1 year, 5.6% at 2 years, 6.9% at 5 years, and 8.4% at 10 years.[5] An estimated 3% to 8% of patients with metastatic cancer will experience pathologic fractures at some point in their lifetime.[6,7]

In some patients, pathologic fracture may be the presenting symptom and lead to the diagnosis of metastatic cancer. A database study in 2016 found roughly 5% of patients hospitalized with bone metastases first presented with pathologic fractures.[8] Skeletal-related events (SREs)—including pathologic fracture, spinal cord compression, and malignant hypercalcemia—were present at diagnosis in 10% to 23% of breast, lung, and prostate cancers.[9] Pathologic fractures are also associated with increased morbidity and mortality. Patients with metastatic

[a] Department of Orthopaedic Surgery, University of Pennsylvania, 3737 Market Street, 6th Floor, Philadelphia, PA 19104, USA; [b] Hospital of the University of Pennsylvania, 3737 Market Street, 6th Floor, Philadelphia, PA 19104, USA
* Corresponding author.
E-mail address: kendall.masada@pennmedicine.upenn.edu

breast cancer and a pathologic fracture have a 32% increased risk of death compared with those without fracture.[10] In metastatic prostate cancer, SRE led to an increase in 1-year mortality from 4.7 to 6.6.[6] This increase in mortality is likely related to both the biology of cancer as well as complications associated with surgical treatment. Many studies have shown that the prophylactic stabilization of impending long bone fractures results in better patient outcomes including shorter hospital stays,[11] lower health care costs,[12] earlier mobilization,[13,14] and lower morbidity.[6,10,15,16] As such, early identification of bone lesions at risk of fracture and subsequent prophylactic stabilization can improve patient care.

Pathophysiology

Pathologic fractures differ from nonpathologic fractures in location, mechanism of injury, pattern, and healing potential. Pathologic fractures more frequently occur in the common location of metastases (eg, the spine, pelvis, proximal femur, and proximal humerus),[3,4] whereas nonpathologic fractures frequently occur in the long bones (eg, femur, tibia/fibula, radius/ulna) and hand.[17] Bone lesions can either be characterized as blastic, lytic, or mixed based on the lesion's radiographic destruction or production of bone, respectively. Although lytic lesions are at highest risk of fracture, both blastic and lytic lesions reduce the load-bearing capabilities of the bone with altered elastic modulus, compressive strength, and tensile yield strain.[18] The altered mechanics make bone more susceptible to fracturing under lower energy loads than might be expected. Pathologic fractures also differ in their fracture patterns: pathologic fractures typically present with transverse or short oblique fracture patterns as compared with fracture patterns commonly more commonly seen in normal bone under higher loading conditions, such as butterfly fragments or comminution.

Pathologic fractures also exhibit altered physiology that inhibits healing. Metastatic bone lesions have a disorganized bone matrix with an imbalance between osteoblasts and osteoclasts. This imbalance is mediated by several factors produced or induced by the tumor cells: Receptor activator of nuclear factor kappa-B ligand, prostaglandin-E, transforming growth factor-alpha and beta, epidermal growth factor, tumor necrosis factor-alpha, interleukins 1 and 6, parathyroid hormone-related peptide, insulin growth factor, endothelin-1, and platelet-derived growth factors.[19] Healing is also further impaired by adjuvant therapies, such as radiation treatments, which are associated with increased numbers of osteoclasts compared with osteoblasts, disrupted vascular supply, and bone marrow fibrosis.[20] This dual inhibition of normal bone formation results in union rates as low as 35% and subjects patients to the complications of nonunion.[21]

Biopsy Principles

When a pathologic fracture is identified through a lesion of unknown origin, a systematic workup must be performed to determine the diagnosis. Although metastasis is the most common cause of bone lesions in adults older 40 years, an unknown lesion should always be approached with a high level of suspicion for a possible primary bone tumor. Inappropriate or incomplete work-up with a misdiagnosis can have devastating complications including local dissemination or systemic progression. Inaccurate diagnosis can not only require additional treatments but also lead to loss of limb or even premature death.[22–24]

Initial workup should include a thorough history, physical examination, and orthogonal radiographs, both of the fracture site and the involved bone in its entirety. The radiographs should provide insight into the nature of the lesion and the fracture pattern. For an isolated lesion in a patient with no prior diagnosis of cancer, a bone scan and CT of the chest, abdomen, and pelvis should be obtained to evaluate for other lesions and a possible primary tumor. A CT of the affected area may also be useful to aid in preoperative planning, especially for pelvic and spine lesions. MRI is indicated to determine the location and extent of primary malignant bone tumors but is not necessary for the evaluation of pathologic fractures related to metastatic disease.

Following imaging, a biopsy is always needed to confirm the diagnosis in the setting of an unknown primary lesion. Biopsies are necessary for any lesion in a patient without a known primary cancer, any solitary lesion in a patient with a known cancer but no history of metastases, and any lesions concerning a primary bone tumor on imaging. Patients with multiple metastases of a biopsy-proven primary cancer do not require biopsy. The goal of the biopsy is to obtain diagnostic tissue in the least invasive manner possible while avoiding contamination or complicating future planned procedures. Improper biopsy technique can result in altered patient outcomes in 8.5% to 10.1% of cases with a 4.5% to 5.5% rate of potentially avoidable amputation.[25,26] Appropriate biopsy requires adherence to the following guiding principles:[27,28]

- The biopsy track is considered contaminated and, in cases of primary bone tumors, will need to be resected with the tumor. Therefore, the incision should be made longitudinally and in line with the planned incision for definitive surgical resection.
- Care should be taken to avoid creating unnecessary tissue planes and to limit exposure to neurovascular structures and uninvolved muscles.
- Strict hemostasis should be maintained, as bleeding or hematoma can contaminate surrounding tissues.
- If a drain is needed to prevent hematoma formation, it should be placed to exit in line with the future surgical resection incision so that it can also be excised during the definitive surgery.
- When possible, the biopsy should be performed by an experienced multidisciplinary sarcoma team, as the risk of complications for a biopsy performed by a nontertiary sarcoma team is five times greater than a biopsy performed by a dedicated sarcoma team.[25,26]

There are 3 different types of biopsies: fine-needle aspiration (FNA), core-needle biopsy, and open biopsy. FNA is not reliable in solid tumors such as sarcomas, because these samples demonstrate cytology but cannot accurately characterize the histologic structure. Historically, the gold standard for bone biopsies is open surgical biopsy because larger tissue samples can be obtained.[29] However, studies have demonstrated similar diagnostic accuracy for percutaneous biopsy with low misdiagnosis rates (3%).[30,31] In addition, image-guided core needle biopsy is often preferred to incisional biopsy given lower risk of complications (0%–10% vs up to 16%), decreased contamination of surrounding tissue, and lower costs.[25,26,29] Finally, percutaneous, image-guided biopsy can be used to target areas of the tumor that seem radiographically suspicious. The type of biopsy modality should ultimately be a shared decision between surgeon and interventional radiology team with the goal of accurate diagnosis and minimal morbidity.

Surgical Treatment

The treatment of pathologic fractures relies on many of the same techniques as fractures in disease-free bone; however, there are important differences as well. Communication with medical oncology to understand the prognosis of the patient is critical. Patients with metastatic cancer are late-stage by definition; while some have short life expectancies and multiple medical comorbidities, others may live for a decade or longer. Patients in advanced stages of disease may prefer nonoperative management of their fractures to avoid the associated morbidity and mortality of surgery. More commonly, surgery is indicated to relieve pain and restore function. In these situations, the focus should be on optimizing short-term rather than long-term outcomes; for example, it is preferable to achieve immediate stability using metal and cement-based constructs than longevity with a biologic reconstruction that will require either a prolonged recovery or carry a risk of early failure. The patient's prognosis and risks, as well as their personal goals and priorities, should be weighed in deciding whether to proceed with surgery and what operation to perform.

The timing of surgery is also an important consideration. Although traditional fracture management recommends expeditious fixation, surgery may need to be delayed in patients with pathologic fractures. Patients without known osseous metastases require a workup, as described previously. Those with an established diagnosis may be undergoing chemotherapy, which would ideally be completed or held before surgery. In general, femur fractures are fixed as soon as possible (ie, within days), whereas fractures in locations such as the humerus, tibia, or acetabulum can be deferred until the patient is optimized (ie, within weeks). Coordination with the medical and radiation oncology teams is thus essential in determining the timing of surgery.

The technical goals of pathologic fracture surgery remain the same as for nonpathologic fracture fixation: restoration of limb length, alignment, and rotation. In addition, emphasis should be placed on early return to weight bearing, attention to impaired bone biology and healing, as well as longevity of the construct appropriate for the patient's life expectancy. Additional fixation strategies such as locking plates/screws and incorporation of polymethyl methacrylate (PMMA) bone cement should be considered whereby approrpiate.[32,33] Locking plates, commonly used for poor bone quality such as in osteoporotic bone, provide improved fixation and limit screw pullout by functioning as fixed-angle devices.[34] These systems have been used successfully in oncologic reconstructions with hardware failure rates reported as 0% to 8% and union 4.75 months after fixation.[35–37] Of note, locking screw technology is only needed when bone is not sufficiently supportive, so it is not necessary for cement or healthy cortices. The implant itself should bridge the lesion and bypass it by at least 2 cortical widths. Lastly, PMMA is a well-established adjuvant for fixation which may assist by filling large osseous voids, providing axial and rotational stability, and improving the pullout strength of screws.[38–40]

The type of fixation used depends on the lesion and its location. Bone metastases are generally managed with intramedullary nails (IMN), plate and screw constructs (ORIF), and arthroplasty techniques, with advantages and disadvantages to each. IMNs offer smaller incisions, stabilization of the entire affected bone, and immediate weight bearing. Although highly effective for long bone diaphyseal lesions, they are not appropriate for most periarticular tumors. Open approaches for ORIF provide direct visualization of the tumor for curettage, reduction, and cement application; however, they require larger incisions and soft tissue dissection with a more limited ability to prophylactically protect the whole affected bone. When applied in conjunction with curettage and cement, they can also support immediate weight-bearing for impending fractures in the lower extremity and impending or completed fractures in the upper extremity. Arthroplasty is also an excellent option, particularly for periarticular lesions. This strategy offers immediate stability independent of healing and reduced risk of local disease progression, but can sometimes involve a more extensive surgery in terms of dissection, operative time, and blood loss, as well as bearing an increased risk of infection.[41,42]

In general, epiphyseal and articular fractures are treated via prosthesis, metaphyseal fractures via plate or prosthesis, and diaphyseal via plate or IMN.[32,42,43] Curettage and PMMA is most common with plating but can also be performed in conjunction with IMNs. Fixation options for the 2 most commonly affected bones in the appendicular skeleton, the humerus and the femur, are outlined later in discussion. Of note, these should be considered guidelines only, as each fracture requires an individualized approach.

Humerus

- Humeral head: Shoulder replacement with hemiarthroplasty, total shoulder arthroplasty, reverse total shoulder arthroplasty, or proximal humerus replacement.
- Surgical neck to the proximal-third shaft: Plate or IMN.

- Diaphysis: IMN or plate.
- Distal: Parallel plating or distal humeral replacement with total elbow arthroplasty.

Femur

- Femoral head and neck: Hemiarthroplasty or total hip arthroplasty.
- Intertrochanteric or subtrochanteric: IMN, calcar-replacing arthroplasty (hemi vs total), or proximal femoral replacement (hemi vs total).
- Diaphyseal: IMN or plate.
- Distal third: plate, IMN, distal femoral replacement.

Adjuvant treatments

Management of pathologic fractures also relies on adjuvant treatments, such as chemotherapy, radiation, bisphosphonates, and embolization, to treat the primary tumor and reduce disease progression.

Chemotherapy

The need for chemotherapy depends on the primary tumor. If given preoperatively, cytotoxic chemotherapy should be held one to 2 weeks before surgery to allow blood counts to recover. Glucocorticoids should be reduced or tapered before surgery to optimize wound healing.[44] Most immunotherapies can be continued perioperatively.[45] There are no definitive recommendations for hormone therapy; however, the increased risk of venous thromboembolisms warrants consideration.[46] Postoperatively cytotoxic chemotherapy and glucocorticoids should be held for approximately 2 weeks until the incision is healed. Any adjustments to a patient's chemotherapy regimen should be discussed first with the patient's medical oncology team.

Radiation Therapy

Radiation therapy, like chemotherapy, may be administered pre or postoperatively for radiation-sensitive cancers. For metastatic disease, radiation is typically used for pain control rather than control of local disease. Preoperative radiation is generally chosen for cases requiring improved pain control, reduction in the size of the lesions, and decreased likelihood of tumor seeding during surgery. Postoperative radiation may also be chosen for pain control and to reduce the rate of local disease progression. Therapy is typically started 2 to 4 weeks after surgery to allow for soft tissue healing.[47] Radiation can also be used as a palliative pain relief measure for patients who are too ill to undergo surgery.

There is a lack of definitive consensus regarding the timing of radiation therapy management of pathologic fractures. The American Society for Therapeutic Radiology and Oncology does not offer guidelines for timing, but does support the use of radiation therapy for pain control with metastases.[48] The conflicting evidence and guidelines emphasize the importance of discussion with the patient's medical and radiation oncology teams to individualize decision-making.

Bisphosphonates

Bisphosphonates, which inhibit osteoclastic bone resorption, can provide another adjunct for managing osseous metastases. Their mechanism of action addresses the underlying imbalance between osteoblast-mediated bone formation and osteoclast-mediated bone resorption seen in pathologic fractures.[49] Bisphosphonates alone have shown some improvement in pain relief of bony metastases in 1 out of 6 patients treated, but there is insufficient evidence to support their use as first-line therapy.[50]

When used in conjunction with radiation therapy, bisphosphonates can reduce skeletal-related events from bony metastases.[51] After the stabilization of complete or impending pathologic fractures, bisphosphonates and radiation therapy can also reduce local tumor progression and improve pain.[52] Timing of bisphosphonate administration is usually begun 2-weeks postoperatively, which has not been shown to delay radiographic or clinical healing.[53]

Embolization

Some hyper-vascular metastatic tumors, such as renal, thyroid, and hepatocellular cancer, may require preoperative embolization. The goal of embolization is to devascularize the tumor before surgical resection, which helps reduce intraoperative blood loss and need for transfusions.[54] Embolization is successful in up to 75% of cases and can obliterate greater than 70% of a tumor's vascularity before surgery. Generally, patients should proceed to surgery within 48 to 72 hours after embolization, before revascularization begins to occur.[55]

Complications

Complications of surgical fixation of pathologic fractures include local progression, nonunion, hardware failure, infections, venous thromboembolisms (VTEs), and bone cement implantation syndrome (BCIS).

Local Progression

Tumor resection can be an important part of strategies designed to reduce local progression in the management of pathologic fractures. The overall rate of local progression can approach 25% but is tumor- and location-dependent.[56] For example, renal cell cancer is relatively resistant to chemotherapy and radiation; it also tends to be expansile with a soft tissue component and highly vascular. One study investigating the intramedullary fixation of pathologic fractures showed renal cell cancer, in addition to age, was an independent risk factor associated with disease progression.[57] For these reasons, while other cancers can be managed with intralesional stabilization and radiation, renal cell metastases may require more aggressive management, such as wide resection, to achieve recurrence-free survival.[33] As such, surgical management of pathologic fractures secondary to renal cell metastases often favors resection and replacement over bony fixation.

Hardware Failure and Nonunion

Pathologic bone exhibits impaired healing resulting in high rates of nonunion and hardware failure. Though data are limited, union rate after metastatic pathologic fracture has been reported as low as 35%.[20] Healing can be further inhibited by chemo or radiation therapy. Chemotherapy causes bone marrow suppression, reducing the number of myeloid cells, and radiation therapy inhibits chondrogenesis. Both cell types are prerequisites for fracture healing.[58] Nonunions place greater strain on the hardware and can lead to early implant failure. One study of patients with femoral metastases who underwent intramedullary nailing for impending or complete pathologic fractures found implant breakage occurred in 8%. Factors associated with implant failure were complete pathologic fractures and prior radiation therapy.[59] A study of pathologic fractures owing to multiple myeloma found hardware failure occurred in 12.5% of cases, all of which occurred outside of the radiation field. This detail suggests that another risk factor for failure may be not including the full operative bed and implant in the radiation field.[60]

The decision to stabilize (ie, with an intramedullary device or plate) versus reconstruct (ie, resect and replace with an endoprosthesis) a metastatic lesion is based on many factors, including tumor histology, size, and location, as well as patient characteristics. A large number of variables limit research on this topic, with only a small case series comparing intramedullary stabilization to endoprosthetic reconstruction.[61] Reconstruction is typically more invasive and carries the risk for arthroplasty-related complications such as infection, dislocation, and aseptic loosening; however, advantages include improved local control and no potential for nonunion. Although osteosynthesis using long plates combined with intramedullary fixation has gained popularity in trauma practices, the success of this technique depends on the healing potential of the bone, making it less useful in treating pathologic fractures for the reasons described above. If nonunion occurs, resection and reconstruction with an endoprosthesis (either arthroplasty or intercalary) are preferred over repeated attempts to achieve fracture healing.

Infections

Postoperative infection is a significant concern, with an incidence as high as 10% to 15% in orthopedic oncology patients.[62] This elevated risk is owing to several factors including patient and surgery characteristics. Patients with cancer can exhibit impaired healing owing to chemotherapy-induced immunodeficiency and/or poor soft tissues owing to radiation, as well as other comorbidities such as diabetes, obesity, and smoking. The prevalence is also high owing to the long duration of oncologic orthopedic surgeries, large incisions, and areas of potential dead space following tumor resection. Inpatient surgery and blood transfusions have also been associated with increased risks of infections.[62–64]

Optimizing the patient's comorbidities and nutritional status preoperatively, as well as the timing of adjuvant therapy, are important for the prevention of infection. Several drains are commonly used to minimize dead space and fluid collections. Other intraoperative prophylactic strategies range from the use of antibiotic cement and silver-coated prostheses to betadine irrigation and vancomycin powder, but data are limited and no standard of care has been established. As such, the use of these strategies must be extrapolated from the joints' literature as there are little supporting data in the orthopedic oncology literature. Perioperative prophylactic antibiotics are also critical. Unlike the standard clinic practice to administer antibiotics for 24 hours postoperatively, many patients undergoing oncologic surgery are given antibiotics for longer postoperative periods. This practice stems from previous research showing extended postoperative antibiotics could reduce the risk of infection from 13% to 8% in patient undergoing endoprosthetic reconstruction.[64]

More recently, an international randomized controlled trial compared the infection rate of patients undergoing endoprosthetic reconstruction for a primary bone tumor or a soft tissue sarcoma who received one versus 5 days of prophylactic intravenous antibiotics and found no significant difference in infection rate between groups. This study focused only on endoprosthetic reconstruction surgeries and did not evaluate the use of prophylactic oral antibiotics.[65] As such, there are still no generalized guidelines regarding the duration of prophylactic antibiotics for orthopedic oncology patients.

Venous Thromboembolisms

At baseline, patients with cancer are at an increased risk of both arterial (2%–5%) and venous (4%–20%) thrombotic events compared with the general population.[66] Surgery increases this risk, as oncologic patients undergoing a procedure have a twofold higher risk of deep vein thrombosis and threefold higher risk of fatal pulmonary embolism compared with patients without cancer.[67] One study found patients with long-bone metastases who undergo surgery have up to a 6% chance of developing VTE following long bone surgery.[68] These elevated risks are still present even when patients are prophylaxed with a course of low molecular weight heparin (LMWH).[69] Perioperative chemotherapy and reduced mobility can further contribute to these risks, highlighting the importance of anticoagulation for oncologic patients undergoing surgical fixation.[70] Current anticoagulation guidelines from the American Society of Clinical Oncology recommend thromboprophylaxis with a direct oral anticoagulant (DOAC), such as apixaban or rivaroxaban, or LMWH for patients undergoing major cancer surgery. This prophylaxis should start before surgery and continue for at least 7 to 10 days after surgery.[71] There are no specific recommendations between DOACs and LMWH. Although DOACs have a nonsignificant trend toward better efficacy owing to the oral route, LMWH is associated with lower rates of bleeding complications.[72]

Another consideration in the incidence of VTE is the use of tranexamic acid (TXA), an antifibrinolytic agent that may be administered either via IV or topically and has proven efficacious in decreasing perioperative blood loss and need for transfusion in patients with total hip and knee arthroplasty.[73,74] Even in patients with known risk factors for postoperative VTE, such as prior VTE or prothrombotic medical comorbidities, TXA has not been associated with increased risk for postoperative VTE.[75,76] The current literature to support of the use of TXA in orthopedic oncology is much more limited. One single-center retrospective study of patients undergoing endoprosthetic reconstruction showed that patients who received topical TXA had reduced perioperative blood loss and transfusion rates without an increase in VTE occurrences.[77] While these results are promising, additional prospective studies are necessary to fully examine the safety of TXA in oncologic patients.

Bone Cement Implantation Syndrome

Bone cement implantation syndrome (BCIS) is a constellation of symptoms that include hypoxia and hypotension shortly after pressurizing cement within the bone. The pathophysiology is not fully understood, but BCIS has been described more consistently within the hip arthroplasty literature. One study demonstrated that up to 75% of oncologic patients who underwent femoral cemented arthroplasty experienced BCIS. Patients older 60 years who had lung cancer also exhibited an increased risk of BCIS.[78] As cement is often necessary to achieve fixation, surgeons can minimize the risk of BCIS by use of a low-viscosity cement mixed under vacuum without pressurization, lavaging the intramedullary canal before the insertion of prosthesis, using the shortest stem necessary, and inserting the stem slowly.[79,80] Communication with anesthesia colleagues and careful monitoring are also key to the recognition of BCIS and initiation of supportive care when necessary.

Pulmonary complications.

Both intramedullary stabilization and insertion of long cemented stems can lead to pulmonary compromise, especially in patients with poor reserve at baseline. Instrumentation of the canal during nailing increases intramedullary pressure, causing the intravasation of bone marrow content and dissemination into the pulmonary circulation. This disruption of the blood flow through the lungs can result in hypoxia, heart failure, and a systemic inflammatory response.[81] Reaming before nail insertion has been shown to increase intramedullary pressure compared with unreamed nailing. Utilization of long stems in arthroplasty reconstructions can also have this effect, with the added risk of bone cement implantation syndrome (BCIS). The mechanism of BCIS is poorly understood, but the physiologic result can include hypoxia, hypotension, pulmonary hypertension, arrhythmias, and cardiac arrest. Clinically, the effect can range from mild hypoxia and confusion postoperatively to intraoperative death.[82] Lastly, reaming through a metastatic lesion may theoretically seem to promote iatrogenic spread of cancer to the lungs; however, the metastatic process depends more on the biological capability of the cancers cells than their physical distribution. A recent retrospective study demonstrated the surgical fixation of pathologic fractures using IMN does not significantly increase the incidence of new metastatic disease to the lungs compared with arthroplasty and ORIF techniques in pathological fractures secondary to breast, prostate, renal, and lung metastases.[83]

The risk of pulmonary complications can be mitigated by the use of venting, that is, drilling a hole into the distal cortex of the canal, which decreases intramedullary pressure by 50% in cadaveric studies.[84] While venting also has the potential to increase the spread of tumor cells to the surrounding tissues, this very rarely has clinical relevance. Suction devices, such as the Reamer-Irrigator-Aspirator (RIA), also reduce pressure and embolization during reaming, though the benefit is less clear. A prospective, multi-center trial examining the use of the RIA in the fixation of isolated nonpathologic femur fractures demonstrated a modest reduction of embolic debris during the reaming and nail insertion segments of the operative procedure in patients who underwent nailing with a RIA; however, the study was unable to correlate that reduction with any changes in physiologic clinical measures.[85] Most importantly, gentle reaming, slow implant insertion, and careful communication with anesthesia are critical to minimize the risk of cardiopulmonary compromise.

SUMMARY

Surgical management of pathologic fractures requires an accurate diagnosis of primary malignancy, which often involves a biopsy. Although the most common cause is metastatic disease, the possibility of a primary bone tumor should always be considered. Pathologic fractures have impaired healing potential with high rates of nonunion and hardware failure. The surgical plan should, therefore, include additional fixation strategies to mitigate these risks and may include locking plate systems, PMMA cement, and arthroplasty. Adjuvant therapy, such as chemotherapy and radiation, may also be used whereby appropriate to reduce local recurrence and improve pain. Optimizing treatment involves the careful coordination of a multidisciplinary team.

CLINICS CARE POINTS

- Accurate diagnosis of the primary malignancy resulting in a pathologic fracture is essential before surgical fixation. The most common cause in adults older 40 years is metastatic disease.
- Diagnosis usually requires biopsy, which should adhere to strict technique guidelines to avoid adverse patient outcomes.
- Pathologic bone has impaired healing and requires additional fixation strategies, such as PMMA cement.
- Adjuvant treatments, such as chemotherapy and radiation, should be coordinated by the medical and radiation oncology teams, respectively.
- Patients with pathologic fractures are at increased risk of postoperative complications compared with those with nonpathologic fractures.

DISCLOSURE

K.M. Masada: None. S.R. Blumenthal: None. C.A. Cipriano: American Association of Hip and Knee Surgeons: Board or committee member. DePuy, A Johnson & Johnson Company: Paid consultant. Musculoskeletal Tumor Society: Board or committee member. Ruth Jackson Orthopedic Society: Board or committee member.

REFERENCES

1. Biermann JS, Holt GE, Lewis VO, et al. Metastatic bone disease: diagnosis, evaluation, and treatment. J Bone Joint Surg Am 2009;91(6):1518–30. PMID: 19487533.
2. American Cancer Society. Cancer facts & figures 2022. Atlanta (GA): American Cancer Society; 2022.
3. Jayarangaiah A, Kemp AK, Theetha Kariyanna P. Bone metastasis. In: StatPearls [internet]. Treasure Island (FL): StatPearls Publishing; 2022. Available at: https://www.ncbi.nlm.nih.gov/books/NBK507911/.
4. Rizzo SE, Kenan S. Pathologic fractures. In: StatPearls [internet]. Treasure Island (FL): StatPearls Publishing; 2022. Available at: https://www.ncbi.nlm.nih.gov/books/NBK559077/.
5. Hernandez RK, Wade SW, Reich A, et al. Incidence of bone metastases in patients with solid tumors: analysis of oncology electronic medical records in the United States. BMC Cancer 2018;18(1):44.
6. Nørgaard M, Jensen AØ, Jacobsen JB, et al. Skeletal related events, bone metastasis and survival of prostate cancer: a population based cohort study in Denmark (1999 to 2007). J Urol 2010;184(1):162–7.
7. Higinbotham NL, Marcove RC. The management of pathological fractures. J Trauma 1965;5(6):792–8. PMID: 5851126.
8. Jairam V, Lee V, Yu JB, et al. Nationwide Patterns of Pathologic Fractures Among Patients Hospitalized With Bone Metastases. Am J Clin Oncol 2020;43(10):720–6.
9. Oster G, Lamerato L, Glass AG, et al. Natural history of skeletal-related events in patients with breast, lung, or prostate cancer and metastases to bone: a 15-year study in two large US health systems. Support Care Cancer 2013;21(12):3279–86.
10. Saad F, Lipton A, Cook R, et al. Pathologic fractures correlate with reduced survival in patients with malignant bone disease. Cancer 2007;110(8):1860–7.
11. El Abiad JM, Raad M, Puvanesarajah V, et al. Prophylactic Versus Postfracture Stabilization for Metastatic Lesions of the Long Bones: A Comparison of 30-day Postoperative Outcomes. J Am Acad Orthop Surg 2019;27(15):e709–16.
12. Blank AT, Lerman DM, Patel NM, et al. Is Prophylactic Intervention More Cost-effective Than the Treatment of Pathologic Fractures in Metastatic Bone Disease? Clin Orthop Relat Res 2016;474(7):1563–70.
13. Arvinius C, Parra JL, Mateo LS, et al. Benefits of early intramedullary nailing in femoral metastases. Int Orthop 2014;38(1):129–32.
14. Ward WG, Holsenbeck S, Dorey FJ, et al. Metastatic disease of the femur: surgical treatment. Clin Orthop Relat Res 2003;415 Suppl:S230–44.
15. Philipp TC, Mikula JD, Doung YC, et al. Is There an Association Between Prophylactic Femur Stabilization and Survival in Patients with Metastatic Bone Disease? Clin Orthop Relat Res 2020;478(3):540–6.
16. Mosher ZA, Patel H, Ewing MA, et al. Early Clinical and Economic Outcomes of Prophylactic and Acute Pathologic Fracture Treatment. J Oncol Pract 2019;15(2):e132–40.
17. GBD 2019 Fracture Collaborators. Global, regional, and national burden of bone fractures in 204 countries and territories, 1990-2019: a systematic analysis from the Global Burden of Disease Study 2019. Lancet Healthy Longev 2021;2(9):e580–92.
18. Kaneko TS, Pejcic MR, Tehranzadeh J, et al. Relationships between material properties and CT scan data of cortical bone with and without metastatic lesions. Med Eng Phys 2003;25(6):445–54.
19. Sekita A, Matsugaki A, Nakano T. Disruption of collagen/apatite alignment impairs bone mechanical function in osteoblastic metastasis induced by prostate cancer. Bone 2017;97:83–93.
20. Pacheco R, Stock H. Effects of radiation on bone. Curr Osteoporos Rep 2013;11(4):299–304.

21. Gainor BJ, Buchert P. Fracture healing in metastatic bone disease. Clin Orthop Relat Res 1983;178:297–302.

22. Adams SC, Potter BK, Mahmood Z, et al. Consequences and prevention of inadvertent internal fixation of primary osseous sarcomas. *Clin Orthop Relat Res* 2009;467(2):519–25.

23. Peabody T. The rodded metastasis is a sarcoma: strategies to prevent inadvertent surgical procedures on primary bone malignancies. Instr Course Lect 2004;53:657–61.

24. Spence GM, Dunning MT, Cannon SR, et al. The hazard of retrograde nailing in pathological fractures: three cases involving primary musculoskeletal malignancy. Injury 2002;33:533–8.

25. Mankin HJ, Mankin CJ, Simon MA. The hazards of the biopsy, revisited. Members of the Musculoskeletal Tumor Society. J Bone Joint Surg Am 1996; 78(5):656–63.

26. Mankin HJ, Lange TA, Spanier SS (2006) THE CLASSIC: The hazards of biopsy in patients with malignant primary bone and soft-tissue tumors. Clin Orthop Relat Res 450:4–10

27. Bickels J, Jelinek JS, Shmookler BM, et al. Biopsy of musculoskeletal tumors. Current concepts. Clin Orthop Relat Res 1999;368:212–9.

28. Traina F, Errani C, Toscano A, et al. Current concepts in the biopsy of musculoskeletal tumors: AAOS exhibit selection. J Bone Joint Surg Am 2015;97(2):e7.

29. Kasraeian S, Allison DC, Ahlmann ER, et al. A comparison of fine-needle aspiration, core biopsy, and surgical biopsy in the diagnosis of extremity soft tissue masses. Clin Orthop Relat Res 2010;468(11):2992–3002.

30. Pohlig F, Kirchhoff C, Lenze U, et al. Percutaneous core needle biopsy versus open biopsy in diagnostics of bone and soft tissue sarcoma: a retrospective study. Eur J Med Res 2012;17(1):29.

31. Adams SC, Potter BK, Pitcher DJ, et al. Office-based core needle biopsy of bone and soft tissue malignancies: an accurate alternative to open biopsy with infrequent complications. Clin Orthop Relat Res 2010;468(10):2774–80.

32. Scolaro JA, Lackman RD. Surgical management of metastatic long bone fractures: principles and techniques. J Am Acad Orthop Surg 2014;22(2):90–100. PMID: 24486755.

33. Arpornsuksant P, Morris CD, Forsberg JA, et al. What Factors Are Associated With Local Metastatic Lesion Progression After Intramedullary Nail Stabilization? Clin Orthop Relat Res 2022;480(5):932–45.

34. Tejwani NC, Guerado E. Improving fixation of the osteoporotic fracture: the role of locked plating. J Orthop Trauma 2011;25(Suppl 2):S56–60.

35. Virkus WW, Miller BJ, Chye PC, et al. The use of locking plates in orthopedic oncology reconstructions. Orthopedics 2008;31(5):438.

36. Gregory JJ, Ockendon M, Cribb GL, et al. The outcome of locking plate fixation for the treatment of periarticular metastases. Acta Orthop Belg 2011; 77(3):362–70.

37. Umer M, Abbas K, Khan S, et al. Locking compression plate in musculoskeletal oncology 'a friend in need. Clin Orthop Surg 2013;5(4):321–6.

38. Cameron HU, Jacob R, Macnab I, et al. Use of polymethylmethacrylate to enhance screw fixation in bone. J Bone Joint Surg Am 1975;57(5):655–6. PMID: 1150708.

39. Wittenberg RH, Lee KS, Shea M, et al. Effect of screw diameter, insertion technique, and bone cement augmentation of pedicular screw fixation strength. Clin Orthop Relat Res 1993;296:278–87. PMID: 8222439.

40. Siegel HJ, Lopez-Ben R, Mann JP, et al. Pathological fractures of the proximal humerus treated with a proximal humeral locking plate and bone cement. J Bone Joint Surg Br 2010;92(5):707–12.

41. Willeumier JJ, van der Linden YM, van de Sande MAJ, et al. Treatment of pathological fractures of the long bones. Open Rev 2017;1(5): 136–45. PMID: 28461940; PMCID: PMC5367617.

42. Kistler BJ, Damron TA. Latest Developments in Surgical and Minimally Invasive Treatment of Metastatic Bone Disease. Curr Surg Rep 2014;2:49.

43. Auran RL, Martin JR, Duran MD, et al. Management of Metastatic Disease in Long Bones. J Orthop Trauma 2022. https://doi.org/10.1097/BOT. 0000000000002360.

44. Wang AS, Armstrong EJ, Armstrong AW. Corticosteroids and wound healing: clinical considerations in the perioperative period. Am J Surg 2013;206(3): 410–7.

45. Elias AW, Kasi PM, Stauffer JA, et al. The Feasibility and Safety of Surgery in Patients Receiving Immune Checkpoint Inhibitors: A Retrospective Study. Front Oncol 2017;7:121.

46. Seim LA, Irizarry-Alvarado JM. Perioperative Management of Female Hormone Medications. Curr Clin Pharmacol 2017;12(3):188–93.

47. Gross CE, Frank RM, Hsu AR, et al. External beam radiation therapy for orthopaedic pathology. J Am Acad Orthop Surg 2015;23(4):243–52.

48. Lutz S, Balboni T, Jones J, et al. Palliative radiation therapy for bone metastases: Update of an ASTRO Evidence-Based Guideline. Pract Radiat Oncol 2017;7(1):4–12.

49. Lin JT, Lane JM. Bisphosphonates. J Am Acad Orthop Surg 2003;11(1):1–4.

50. Wong R, Wiffen PJ. Bisphosphonates for the relief of pain secondary to bone metastases. Cochrane Database Syst Rev 2002;2002(2):CD002068.

51. Al Farii H, Frazer A, Farahdel L, et al. Bisphosphonates Versus Denosumab for Prevention of Pathological Fracture in Advanced Cancers With Bone

Metastasis: A Meta-analysis of Randomized Controlled Trials. J Am Acad Orthop Surg Glob Res Rev 2020;4(8):e2000045.

52. Wolanczyk MJ, Fakhrian K, Adamietz IA. Radiotherapy, Bisphosphonates and Surgical Stabilization of Complete or Impending Pathologic Fractures in Patients with Metastatic Bone Disease. J Cancer 2016;7(1):121–4.

53. Barton DW, Smith CT, Piple AS, et al. Timing of Bisphosphonate Initiation After Fracture: What Does the Data Really Say? Geriatr Orthop Surg Rehabil 2020;11. 2151459320980369.

54. Pazionis TJ, Papanastassiou ID, Maybody M, et al. Embolization of hypervascular bone metastases reduces intraoperative blood loss: a case-control study. Clin Orthop Relat Res 2014;472(10):3179–87.

55. Geraets SEW, Bos PK, van der Stok J. Preoperative embolization in surgical treatment of long bone metastasis: a systematic literature revi. efort Open Rev 2020;5(1):17–25.

56. Healey JH, Brown HK. Complications of bone metastases: surgical management. Cancer 2000;88(12 Suppl):2940–51.

57. Higuchi T, Yamamoto N, Hayashi K, et al. The Efficacy of Wide Resection for Musculoskeletal Metastatic Lesions of Renal Cell Carcinoma. Anticancer Res 2018;38(1):577–82.

58. Coleman RE. Metastatic bone disease: clinical features, pathophysiology and treatment strategies. Cancer Treat Rev 2001;27(3):165–76.

59. Willeumier JJ, Kaynak M, van der Zwaal P, et al. What Factors Are Associated With Implant Breakage and Revision After Intramedullary Nailing for Femoral Metastases? Clin Orthop Relat Res 2018;476(9):1823–33.

60. Elhammali A, Milgrom SA, Amini B, et al. Postoperative Radiotherapy for Multiple Myeloma of Long Bones: Should the Entire Rod Be Treated? Clin Lymphoma Myeloma Leuk 2019;19(8):e465–9.

61. Gao H, Liu Z, Wang B, et al. Clinical and functional comparison of endoprosthetic replacement with intramedullary nailing for treating proximal femur metastasis. Chin J Cancer Res 2016;28(2):209–14.

62. Anatone AJ, Danford NC, Jang ES, et al. Risk Factors for Surgical Site Infection in Orthopaedic Oncology. J Am Acad Orthop Surg 2020;28(20):e923–8.

63. Morris CD, Sepkowitz K, Fonshell C, et al. Prospective identification of risk factors for wound infection after lower extremity oncologic surgery. Ann Surg Oncol 2003;10(7):778–82.

64. Donati D, Biscaglia R. The use of antibiotic-impregnated cement in infected reconstructions after resection for bone tumours. J Bone Joint Surg Br 1998;80(6):1045–50.

65. Racano A, Pazionis T, Farrokhyar F, et al. High infection rate outcomes in long-bone tumor surgery with endoprosthetic reconstruction in adults: a systematic review. Clin Orthop Relat Res 2013;471(6):2017–27.

66. Prophylactic Antibiotic Regimens in Tumor Surgery (PARITY) Investigators, Ghert M, Schneider P, Guyatt G, et al. Comparison of Prophylactic Intravenous Antibiotic Regimens After Endoprosthetic Reconstruction for Lower Extremity Bone Tumors: A Randomized Clinical Trial. JAMA Oncol 2022;8(3):345–53.

67. Grover SP, Hisada YM, Kasthuri RS, et al. Cancer Therapy-Associated Thrombosis. Arterioscler Thromb Vasc Biol 2021;41(4):1291–305.

68. Nijziel MR, van Oerle R, Hillen HF, et al. From Trousseau to angiogenesis: the link between the haemostatic system and cancer. Neth J Med 2006;64(11):403–10. PMID: 17179570.

69. Groot OQ, Ogink PT, Janssen SJ, et al. High Risk of Venous Thromboembolism After Surgery for Long Bone Metastases: A Retrospective Study of 682 Patients. Clin Orthop Relat Res 2018;476(10):2052–61.

70. Mioc ML, Prejbeanu R, Vermesan D, et al. Deep vein thrombosis following the treatment of lower limb pathologic bone –ractures - a comparative study. BMC Musculoskelet Disord 2018;19(1):213.

71. Oppelt P, Betbadal A, Nayak L. Approach to chemotherapy-associated thrombosis. Vasc Med 2015;20(2):153–61.

72. Key NS, Khorana AA, Kuderer NM, et al. Venous Thromboembolism Prophylaxis and Treatment in Patients With Cancer: ASCO Clinical Practice Guideline Update. J Clin Oncol 2020;38(5):496–520.

73. The ICM-VTE Oncology Delegates* Recommendations from the ICM-VTE: Oncology. J Bone Joint Surg 2022;104(Suppl 1):232–7.

74. Aguilera X, Martinez-Zapata MJ, Bosch A, et al. Efficacy and safety of fibrin glue and tranexamic acid to prevent postoperative blood loss in total knee arthroplasty: a randomized controlled clinical trial. J Bone Joint Surg Am 2013;95(22):2001–7.

75. Chang CH, Chang Y, Chen DW, et al. Topical tranexamic acid reduces blood loss and transfusion rates associated with primary total hip arthroplasty. Clin Orthop Relat Res 2014;472(5):1552–7.

76. Whiting DR, Gillette BP, Duncan C, et al. Preliminary results suggest tranexamic acid is safe and effective in arthroplasty patients with severe comorbidities. Clin Orthop Relat Res 2014;472(1):66–72.

77. Sabbag OD, Abdel MP, Amundson AW, et al. Tranexamic Acid Was Safe in Arthroplasty Patients With a History of Venous Thromboembolism: A Matched Outcome Study. J Arthroplasty 2017;32(9S):S246–50.

78. Haase DR, Templeton KJ, Rosenthal HG, et al. Tranexamic Acid in Patients With Cancer Undergoing

Endoprosthetic Reconstruction: A Retrospective Review. J Am Acad Orthop Surg 2020;28(6):248–55.

79. Schwarzkopf E, Sachdev R, Flynn J, et al. Occurrence, risk factors, and outcomes of bone cement implantation syndrome after hemi and total hip arthroplasty in cancer patients. J Surg Oncol 2019;120(6):1008–15.

80. Hines CB. Understanding Bone Cement Implantation Syndrome. AANA J 2018;86(6):433–41.

81. Rudloff MI, Smith WR. Intramedullary nailing of the femur: current concepts concerning reaming. J Orthop Trauma 2009;23(5 Suppl):S12–7.

82. Donaldson AJ, Thomson HE, Harper NJ, et al. Bone cement implantation syndrome. Br J Anaesth 2009;102(1):12–22.

83. Hall JA, McKee MD, Vicente MR, et al. Prospective Randomized Clinical Trial Investigating the Effect of the Reamer-Irrigator-Aspirator on the Volume of Embolic Load and Respiratory Function During Intramedullary Nailing of Femoral Shaft Fractures. J Orthop Trauma 2017;31(4):200–4.

84. Roth SE, Rebello MM, Kreder H, et al. Pressurization of the metastatic femur during prophylactic intramedullary nail fixation. J Trauma 2004;57(2):333–9.

85. Kendal JK, Heard BJ, Abbott AG, et al. Does surgical technique influence the burden of lung metastases in patients with pathologic long bone fractures? BMC Musculoskelet Disord 2022;23(1):102.

Pediatrics

Benign Bone Lesions Found in Childhood

Marcos R. Gonzalez, MD[a], Ty K. Subhawong, MD[b], Juan Pretell-Mazzini, MD[c],*

KEYWORDS

- Bone tumor • Benign • Epidemiology • Diagnosis • Treatment • Recurrence

KEY POINTS

- Benign bone tumors are a diverse group of neoplasms, usually asymptomatic, diagnosed in most cases due to secondary causes.
- Plain radiographs are always the first imaging tool employed and in most cases are enough to reach a diagnosis. CT scan and MRI can help in cases of equivocal lesions. Biopsy is not commonly required.
- Treatment approach depends on a correct assessment of the lesion's risk of progression, development of secondary malignancy, and the patient's symptoms. In the majority of cases, expectant treatment is the first line.
- When interventional treatment is mandatory, treatment options include minimally invasive methods and surgery. Recurrence rates for each procedure and the surgeon's expertise determine the optimal approach.

INTRODUCTION

Benign bone tumors represent a varied array of neoplasms that often arise during childhood. Tumors belonging to this group show different frequency rates, clinical manifestations, and treatment approaches. Indeed, the real incidence of benign bone tumors in children is not known, as many tumors are silent.

Large retrospective databases show cartilaginous tumors as the most common type of benign bone lesion, consisting primarily of osteochondromas and enchondromas.[1] However, additional studies indicate that the incidence in children of fibrous cortical defects, mainly nonossifying fibromas (NOF), is between 30% and 40%.[2] Due to the characteristic radiographic features and known spontaneous resolution of NOF, a biopsy is not often requested and they are, therefore, underestimated in biopsy-driven bone tumor databases.

Most benign bone tumors are asymptomatic and incidentally discovered only after a radiograph is taken due to a recent injury or other secondary causes. A smaller group of patients may present with a history of pain, palpable mass, or pathologic fracture. Furthermore, there is not a single pathognomonic presentation of all benign bone tumors; rather, tumors may show typical patterns that set them apart from the group, as it occurs in the case of osteoid osteomas.

Plain radiographs are the first imaging tool employed when a benign bone tumor is suspected. Features such as tumor location (flat or long bone), segment of bone involved (epiphysis, diaphysis, metaphysis), and radiographic features of the lesion may be useful for 2 purposes: (1) narrow down the differential diagnosis or establish the diagnosis, and (2) determine the likely growth rate and aggressiveness of the

[a] Facultad de Medicina Alberto Hurtado, Universidad Peruana Cayetano Heredia, Av. Honorio Delgado 430, Urb Ingenieria, San Martin de Porres, Lima- Peru; [b] Department of Radiology, Division of Musculoskeletal Radiology, University of Miami Miller School of Medicine, 1611 NW 12th avenue, Miami, FL 33136, USA; [c] Division of Orthopedic Oncology, Miami Cancer Institute, Baptist Health System South Florida, 1228 South Pine Island Road, Suite 410. Plantation, FL 33324, USA
* Corresponding author. Miami Cancer Institute – Plantation, FL 333324.
E-mail address: juan.pretell@baptisthealth.net

Orthop Clin N Am 54 (2023) 59–74
https://doi.org/10.1016/j.ocl.2022.08.001

tumor. In 1980, Lodwick and colleagues[3] established an algorithm to determine the growth rate of a lytic bone lesion (Table 1). The importance of growth rates stems from their considerable accuracy in correlating with malignancy.

Plain radiographs through 2 orthogonal planes are also employed for the staging of benign bone tumors. The Enneking staging system, first published in the 1980s and subsequently adopted by the Musculoskeletal Tumor Society (MSTS), classified benign bone tumors as latent benign (stage 1), active benign (stage 2), and aggressive benign (stage 3).[4] According to the tumor stage, he established levels of surgical margins and indicated if adjuvant therapy was required to minimize tumor recurrence.

Despite the widespread use of radiographs in children with bone tumors, lytic lesions are often not detected until a 30–50% loss of mineralization has occurred.[5] Therefore, complementary imaging tools such as computed tomography (CT), magnetic resonance imaging (MRI) and skeletal scintigraphy (bone scan) are often employed.

BENIGN OSSEOUS TUMORS: OSTEOCHONDROMA, OSTEOID OSTEOMA, AND OSTEOBLASTOMA

Osteochondroma is the most common benign bone tumor, constituting 20–50% of all benign tumors and 10–15% of all bone tumors.[6] Similar to other benign bone tumors, its incidence is unknown as most cases are asymptomatic. Osteochondromas are composed of both cortical and medullary bone covered by a cartilaginous cap. Most of them are isolated, but a minority of patients may develop multiple lesions as part of a genetic disease. Multiple hereditary exostoses (MHE) is an autosomal dominant disease characterized by the development of multiple osteochondromas and a much higher risk of malignant transformation.

Osteochondromas are typically located around the knee, with most lesions in the proximal tibia (28%), distal femur (18%), and proximal humerus (8%).[7] These tumors usually involve the metaphysis of long bones, and when patients achieve skeletal maturity, rate of growth diminishes or ceases altogether.

Osteochondromas are usually asymptomatic and found on incidental imaging. When they cause pain, it is usually due to compromise of adjacent structures, fracture, or malignant transformation.[8] When symptomatic, it may cause referred pain, paresthesia, loss of pulse, and/or changes in the color of feet due to compromise

of surrounding structures or a palpable mass in the case of a pedunculated osteochondroma.

The most feared complication of osteochondromas is malignant transformation. Rates fluctuate between 1% for single osteochondroma and 10% for HME.[8]

Osteoid osteoma is the third most common benign bone tumor. Its incidence is 11% among benign bone tumors and 3% among all bone tumors.[9] It usually affects patients < 30 years old and has a peak incidence during the second and third decade of life.[10] Lesions are usually located in the lower limbs, with the proximal femur being the most common location; spinal compromise occurs in 6–20% of patients.[11] Patients typically present with weeks to months history of dull pain, which aggravates at night and is relieved with nonsteroidal anti-inflammatory drugs (NSAIDs).[12]

Osteoblastomas commonly occur in people younger than 40, with the highest incidence between 10 and 25 years.[13] The most commonly affected areas include the axial skeleton (33%), craniofacial bones (16%), and the hands and feet (14%).[13,14] They usually do not show a characteristic pattern of pain as osteoid osteomas; rather, most patients present with a long history of dull pain that does not improve with NSAIDs and does not worsen at night.

Radiological findings

Osteochondromas are often diagnosed only with radiographs, especially when the metaphysis is compromised.[15] The lesions consist of cortical and medullary bone emerging from the surface of the bone, often in the shape of a stalk or flat protuberance (Fig. 1A). Additional findings include multiple calcifications within the cartilaginous component of the osteochondroma, seen as radiopaque, and bone degeneration under the affected bone cortex, seen as radiolucent.[16]

Continuous growth of an osteochondroma after growth plate closure, irregular or lobulated margin, irregular or scattered calcifications, internal lytic areas, and erosion or destruction of adjacent bones raise are features that may indicate risk of malignant transformation, typically a secondary chondrosarcoma.[8] Furthermore, new onset of pain in an area with a preexisting osteochondroma should warrant further imaging, usually an MRI. On MRI, a cartilage cap thickness exceeding 2 cm in adults and 3 cm in children should raise the suspicion of malignant transformation (Fig. 1B).[17]

In patients with suspicion of an osteoid osteoma, characteristic clinical presentation and

Table 1
Lodwick's system to grade bone destruction according to radiographic features

Radiographic Pattern	IA	IB	IC	II	III
Destruction	Geographic (Mandatory)	Geographic (Mandatory)	Geographic (Mandatory)	Moth-eaten or Geographic	Permeated (Mandatory)
Edge characteristic	(One of the 3 patterns) Regular (1) Lobulated (2) Multicentric (3)	(One of the 4 patterns) Regular (1) Lobulated (2) Multicentric (3) Ragged/poorly defined (4)	(One of the 5 patterns) Regular (1) Lobulated (2) Multicentric (3) Ragged/poorly defined (4) Moth-eaten, 1 cm or less (5)	If Geographic, mandatory moth-eaten edge greater than 1 cm	Any edge
Penetration of cortex	None or partial	None or partial	Mandatory total	Total by definition	Total by definition
Sclerotic rim	Mandatory	Optional	Optional	Optional but unlikely	Optional but unlikely
Expanded shell	Optional only 1 cm or less	If sclerotic rim present, expanded shell must be greater than 1 cm	Optional	Optional but unlikely	Optional but unlikely

Tumors classified as grade I present the lowest growth rate, while those classified as grade III show the highest rate.

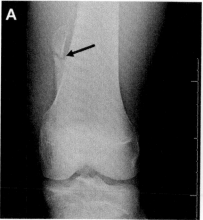 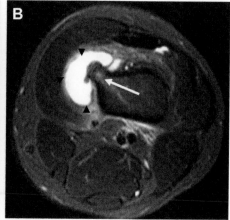

Fig. 1. Fifteen-year-old male with medial left thigh pain. (A) AP radiograph shows a fractured osteochondroma (*arrow*). (B) Axial fat-suppressed proton-density weighted MRI shows corticomedullary continuity of the lesion (*arrow*), a pathognomonic feature of osteochondroma, and surrounding fluid (*arrowheads*) related to adventitious bursitis, hemorrhage, and edema from the fracture.

plain radiographs are sufficient to reach a diagnosis. Classic radiographic features include a round or oval area of cortical thickening and reactive sclerosis containing a radiolucent nidus usually less than 1.5–2 cm (Fig. 2A and B).[18] Jordan and colleagues[19] reported a 66.4% sensitivity of plain radiographs for diagnosing osteoid osteomas in a recent systematic review. Similarly, MRI missed the diagnosis in 34.7% of cases while CT (Fig. 2C and D) proved to be the superior imaging tool with a 96.4% sensitivity. Osteoblastomas appear as radiolucent lesions with surrounding reactive sclerosis on plain radiographs. A significantly larger nidus size (typically > 2 cm) and greater cortical expansion distinguish osteoblastoma from osteoid osteomas.[14] However, radiographs are not completely reliable to differentiate osteoblastoma from malignant lesions. We recommend doing a CT scan in all patients with suspected osteoblastomas to provide better detail about the nature of the tumor.

Treatment

In the case of an asymptomatic isolated osteochondroma, surgery is not indicated as the risk of malignant transformation is extremely low. Indications for surgical treatment include unremitting pain, cosmetic reasons, and/or increased risk of malignant transformation. Patients with multiple osteochondromas due to MHE undergo surgical treatment more often due to higher risk of malignant transformation and more lesions that become symptomatic.

When surgery is indicated, complete resection of the osteochondroma at the normal bone base is recommended. To minimize the risks of recurrence, the perichondrium and cartilage cap should be completely removed. In the case of children, tumor resection might be delayed until skeletal maturity is attained due to a probable higher relapse rate.[20] In addition, surgeons must be extremely careful when the lesion is located close to the growth plate to avoid damage.

The initial treatment of osteoid osteomas is initially conservative with NSAIDs due to their self-limited course and ability to regress spontaneously. Patients who do not respond to NSAIDs or do not tolerate their prolonged use are candidates for invasive management. Despite its high success rate, surgical treatment has been progressively replaced by minimally invasive techniques due to lower complication rates and similar efficacy. A recent systematic review by Lindquester and colleagues[21] found no significant difference in the efficacy of osteoid osteoma treatment between radiofrequency and cryoablation, with an overall efficacy of 91.9% (Fig. 2E).

Osteoblastoma must be managed surgically due to its potential local aggressive behavior.[13] Surgical treatment is based on intralesional curettage or *en bloc* resection depending on the case. Intralesional curettage with bone grafting is usually the first line in most patients. *En bloc* resection is typically reserved for locally aggressive tumors or recurrent osteoblastomas after failed curettage. Berry and colleagues followed 99 patients with osteoblastoma treated with either curettage and bone grafting or *en bloc* resection. They reported a local recurrence rate of 23% for curettage and 14% for *en bloc* resection.[22]

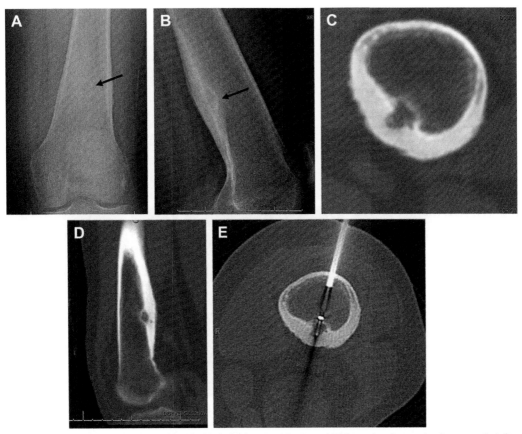

Fig. 2. Twenty-four-year-old male with distal left thigh pain. (A) AP and (B) lateral radiographs show a well-defined radiolucent lesion eccentrically located along the posterior aspect of the distal femoral diaphysis (*arrows*), typical of osteoid osteoma. The associated posterior solid smooth periosteal reaction and cortical thickening indicate indolence. (C) Axial and (D) sagittal CT demonstrate the endosteal radiolucent nidus with few internal punctate calcifications. (E) Intraprocedural axial CT demonstrates the radiofrequency ablation (RFA) probe centered in the nidus.

CARTILAGINOUS TUMORS: CHONDROBLASTOMA, CHONDROMYXOID FIBROMA, AND ENCHONDROMA

Chondroblastomas constitute 1–2% of all primary bone tumors and approximately 5% of benign bone tumors.[23] Although having been reported in all age ranges, most affected patients are aged < 20 years. The most common sites include the proximal femur (20.7%), distal femur (18.5%), proximal tibia (16.3%), proximal humerus (12%), and foot (10.9%).[24]

Chondroblastoma typically presents insidiously, with patients typically reporting pain lasting for months to years. Pain with local tenderness in the involved bone and adjacent joint is the most common clinical presentation, followed by decreased range of motion.[25] In patients with suspected chondroblastoma of the foot, a subchondral fracture is common and painful, and is not always obvious on plain radiographs.[26]

Chondromyxoid fibroma (CMF) is another infrequent benign tumor that occurs in < 0.5% of all bone tumors.[27] This tumor usually affects young patients in their second and third decade of life, with 72% of affected patients being < 40 years of age.[28] About half of the lesions are found in the appendicular skeleton, including tibia (55.4%), followed by the femur (19.2%) and fibula (10.8%). Lesions in the flat bones and bones of the hands and feet are also found in 30.3% and 17.3% of cases, respectively.[28] Patients with CMF often present with a long history of intermittent pain that does not cause significant distress.

Enchondromas are much less common than chondroblastomas, representing only 2.6% of all benign bone tumors. Mostly asymptomatic, they can present at any age although most commonly between the first and fourth decade

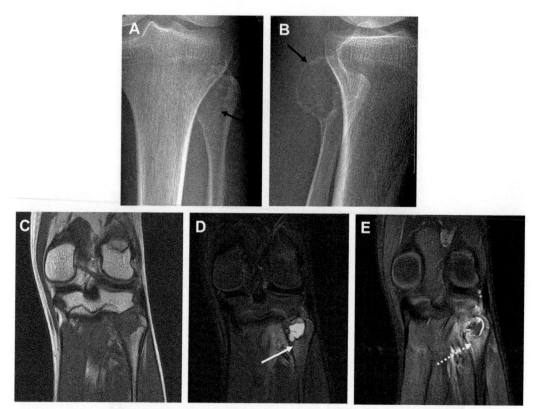

Fig. 3. Fifteen-year-old male with proximal left leg pain. (*A*) AP and (*B*) lateral radiographs demonstrate an expansile lytic lesion in the fibular head (*arrows*). (*C*) Coronal T1-weighted, (*D*) coronal fat-suppressed proton-density weighted and (*E*) coronal fat-suppressed contrast-enhanced MRI highlight the lobular morphology of the epiphyseal lesion centered in the epiphysis, with perilesional bone marrow edema (*arrow* in D) and enhancement (*dashed arrow* in E), typical of chondroblastoma.

of life.[29] They are usually located in the short tubular bones of the hands but can occasionally be found in the long bones.[30] Enchondromas are usually found as solitary lesions but may rarely appear as multiple lesions, as part of a condition known as multiple enchondromatosis.

Radiological findings

The classic radiographic appearance of chondroblastomas is sharply defined lytic round or oval lesion, eccentrically located in the bone epiphysis next to an open growth plate (Fig. 3A and B).[25] Most lesions are < 4 cm in diameter and fine intralesional calcifications can be found, especially in skeletally immature patients. Although located in the epiphysis, metaphyseal invasion is not uncommon and has been reported to occur in up to 58% of cases.[31] In contrast, pure metaphyseal or diaphyseal lesions are extremely rare and occur in 1.8% of cases. A small number of chondroblastomas present in conjunction with an aneurysmal bone cyst (ABC), which distorts common lesion radiographic parameters and makes diagnosis harder.

CT scans help determine the distance between the lesion and the physis ~~growth plate~~, important for preoperative planning, and the relation of the lesion to the subchondral bone.[32] The latter is extremely important to assess areas such as the foot, where plain radiographs cannot detect subchondral fractures. MRI, when used without prior radiographs, leads to the overestimation of tumor aggressiveness (Fig. 3C–E).[33] Therefore, plain radiographs should antecede more advanced imaging tools such as CT and MRI.

CMF typically presents as a lytic radiolucent medullary lesion located in the metaphyseal region.[27] The tumor shows a scalloped border with a well-defined thin rim of sclerotic bone (Fig. 4). In small bones, CMF tends to occupy the entire width of the bone and causes thinning of the cortices.[32] The tumor shows "pseudotrabeculations," which are the ridges of the sclerotic rim at the edge of the lesion.[27] In addition, the absence of calcifications on imaging serves as an important diagnostic clue to differentiate CMF from other cartilaginous

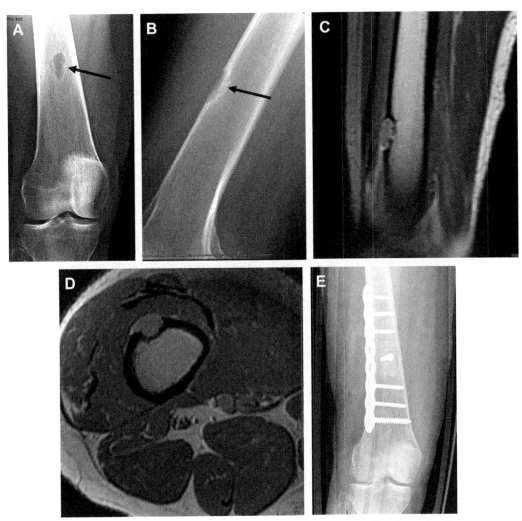

Fig. 4. Fifty-one-year-old female with right thigh pain. (A) AP and (B) lateral radiographs show an eccentric geographic lytic lesion in the femoral diaphysis, with well-defined sclerotic margins. (C) Sagittal and (D) axial proton-density weighted MRI shows the cortically based lesion, without intramedullary involvement. (E) AP radiograph status postexcision of the chondromyxoid fibroma with allograft reconstruction and lateral plate and screw fixation.

tumors. In fact, the radiographic prevalence of calcifications in this tumor has been reported at 2.5% to 12.5%, much lower than in other cartilaginous tumors.[27,34] As in chondroblastoma, CT and MRI are the preferred imaging techniques for CMF. CT scans help assess the integrity of the cortices and MRI can help with staging and preoperative planning.

Enchondromas usually appear on plain radiographs as well-defined lytic and slightly expansile lesion. On plain radiographs, they show stippled calcifications without or mild endosteal scalloping.[30] Additional imaging techniques such as CT and MRI are required to identify additional features of malignancy such as deep endosteal scalloping, cortical destruction, and soft tissue mass as well as periosteal reaction. Murphey and colleagues[35] reported that endosteal scalloping of more than two-thirds of the cortical thickness had excellent discriminating ability; 75% of chondrosarcomas fulfilled this criterion, in contrast to only 9% of enchondromas.

Treatment

Chondroblastomas are surgically treated as there is no evidence of potential spontaneous healing and there is no available medical treatment. Surgical management consists of curettage and bone grafting.[36] To avoid damaging the epiphyseal growth plate, the use of intraoperative imaging is often employed. Furthermore, Lin and colleagues reported that an open growth plate did not compromise the ability to perform a thorough curettage and found lower recurrence rates among patients aged < 16 years. They also reported no significant difference in recurrence rates between curettage and en bloc resection.[36] Known risk factors for recurrence include the location of the tumor in the pelvis and strictly epiphyseal lesions.[36,37]

After curettage, bone graft is the preferred material to fill the cavitary defect although polymethyl methacrylate (PMMA) is also often employed. Adjuvant therapy is not indicated due to insufficient evidence supporting its benefits.[38]

Management of chondromyxoid fibroma consists of curettage or resection, both with and without filling the cavity. Although wide or en bloc resection achieves the lowest recurrence, it is not always indicated the first line due to higher rate of associated complications. Lersundi and colleagues reported a 38% recurrence rate among patients with chondromyxoid fibroma treated with curettage alone. The rate diminished to 13% and 0% in patients treated with adjuvant therapy. The rate of recurrence in patients who underwent curettage + PMMA was similar to the one in patients treated with resection.[39]

Enchondromas are usually treated nonoperatively unless they are symptomatic, actively enlarging or there is an impending fracture.[30] When surgical management is indicated, treatment consists of intralesional excision followed by filling the defect with bone graft or PMMA. Due to its low recurrence, the use of adjuvant treatments is not normally necessary.

FIBROUS LESIONS: NONOSSIFYING FIBROMA AND FIBROUS DYSPLASIA

Nonossifying fibroma (NOF) is a common benign bone lesion that commonly affects children younger than 15 years. It is estimated that NOFs affect approximately 30–40% of all pediatric patients.[40] NOFs are part of a disease spectrum that also includes fibrous cortical defects (FCDs) and the Jaffe–Campanacci syndrome.[41] FCDs are smaller, asymptomatic lesions often found on incidental radiographs that tend to spontaneously heal. When these lesions attain proliferative activity and significantly increase in size, they are called NOF.[42] Multiple NOFs may also present in association with café-au-lait spots and axillary freckling and are classified as the Jaffe–Campanacci syndrome.[41]

Currently, NOFs are considered an alteration of normal metaphyseal remodeling rather than a true neoplastic process. In the majority of cases, these lesions stop proliferating once skeletal maturity is attained and gradual reossification eventually leads to their spontaneous resolution.[43]

NOF are typically asymptomatic and found during incidental imaging due to other reasons. Lesions are typically metaphyseal and most commonly located on the distal femur, proximal tibia, distal tibia, proximal humerus, fibula and radius.[41] When symptomatic, they may cause swelling and pain, often associated with movement. Physicians should pay close attention to patients complaining of persistent pain, as it may indicate the risk for pathologic fracture.[40]

Fibrous dysplasia (FD) is the second most common fibrous abnormality found in the bone, accounting for approximately 5% to 7% of all benign bone tumors.[44] FD is considered a postzygotic mutation in the GNAS1 gene.[45] This results in a failed bone realignment response after mechanical stress and the inability to remodel primitive bone into lamellar bone.[44]

FD can affect a single bone (monostotic) or multiple bones (polyostotic) and be associated with the compromise of other organs. Monostotic disease represents around 70% of FD cases and typically presents during the third decade of life, while polyostotic disease presents in the first decade.[46] In decreasing order of frequency, monostotic FD affects the craniofacial bones, ribs, and femur, while polyostotic disease most often located in the femur, tibia, and skull and facial bones. Unlike monostotic lesions, which are typically asymptomatic and present as an incidental finding, 60% of patients with polyostotic FD present symptoms before the age of 10. The most common symptoms are pain and spontaneous fracture.[46]

In 3% of patients, bone lesions present together with skin pigmentation and hyperfunctioning endocrine disorders as part of the McCune–Albright syndrome.[47] Even less frequently, Mazabraud syndrome presents with bone lesions and intramuscular myxomas.[46]

Radiological findings

NOFs have a typical radiographic appearance characterized by a lytic, eccentric, and ovoid lesion classically located in the bone metaphysis.[48] A narrow zone of transition, often with sclerotic borders, is found between the lytic area and the healthy, metaphyseal bone (Fig. 5A).[49] The thin sclerotic rim indicates the slow-growing nature of the lesion, where healthy bone has had time to react and lay down dense

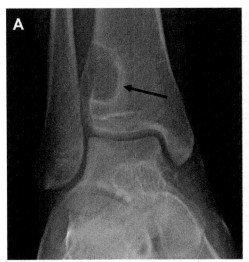 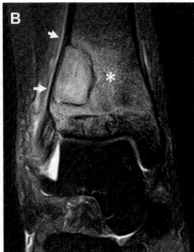

Fig. 5. Sixteen-year-old female with right ankle pain. (*A*) AP radiograph shows an eccentric lytic lesion in the distal aspect of the right tibia, with well-defined sclerotic margins (*arrow*). (*B*) Coronal fat-suppressed proton-density MRI demonstrates significant perilesional bone marrow edema (*), and the presence of periosteal reaction (*short arrows*), atypical findings for nonossifying fibroma but ones that denote ongoing stress reaction and trabecular microfractures, and may signify impending pathologic fracture.

bone adjacent to the lesion.[40] Clinical and radiological features are usually enough to reach diagnosis and biopsy is not commonly required. Diagnosis of atypical lesions may be aided with the use of CT scan or MRI to better visualize the radiological features of NOF (Fig. 5B).[45]

Unlike NOF, the presentation of FD is highly variable. The most common presentation includes a radiolucent lesion, with a grayish "ground-glass" pattern similar to the density of cancellous bone, with no visible trabecular pattern.[50] Despite arising from the medullary canal, lesions typically replace both cancellous and cortical bone and make the distinction between the cortex and canal dimmer.[44] Lesions may also present features such as bony expansion, endosteal scalloping, and a thick reactive bone "rind."

The "shepherd crook" deformity is a pathognomonic finding of FD characterized by the pathological curvature of the femoral neck and proximal femur (Fig. 6). Patients with this feature are at increased risk of pathological fracture and may require surgical intervention.[46]

Additional imaging is often recommended when FD is suspected. Bone scintigraphy helps elucidate the extent of the disease as lesions show increased radiotracer uptake. If monostotic FD is confirmed, physicians should know that progression to polyostotic disease does not occur, lesions do not increase in size over time, and disease becomes inactive at puberty.[50] CT and MRI can provide additional information about soft tissue extension or when the radiographic appearance of the lesion is ambiguous.[51]

Treatment
Treatment of newly diagnosed, asymptomatic NOFs is expectant and consists of radiographic monitoring until the lesion regresses. It is not uncommon for lesions to increase in size and become symptomatic during the growth spurt.

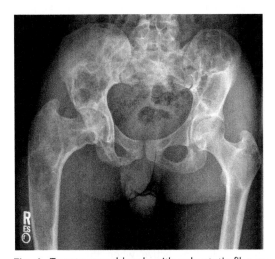

Fig. 6. Twenty-year-old male with polyostotic fibrous dysplasia. AP radiograph shows multiple geographic lytic lesions with well-defined sclerotic borders, throughout the pelvis and both femurs. The resultant intramedullary expansion and cortical remodeling in the right proximal femur have led to a characteristic "shepherd's crook" deformity.

Indications for surgery include persistent pain and high risk of impending fracture. For nonfibular NOF, a lesion occupying more than 50% of the transverse diameter of the affected bone or exceeding 33 mm in its maximum dimension has a high risk of fracture according to Arata's criteria.[42] Orthopedic surgeons should also bear in mind that smaller lesions in high-stress areas such as the distal femoral metaphysis may also be at high risk of fractures, especially among children that engage in contact sports.[45]

Among patients with persistent pain, surgical management consists of curettage and bone grafting. Both autogenous bone and synthetic substitutes can be used to fill the bone defect, depending on the surgeon's and the patient's preferences.[45] Arata and colleagues[42] reported the management of 23 cases of pathological fractures due to NOF and suggested that when the fracture is stable with a hairline fracture through only one cortex, immediate curettage and concomitant autogenous bone-grafting results in the most rapid resolution of the defect. When the lesion is near an actively growing physis, delaying the surgery may decrease the chances of damaging the growth place during curettage and grafting.

FD lesions do not typically progress to pathological fracture and are observed periodically. In the case of polyostotic disease, we recommend referral to an endocrinologist to rule out associated metabolic diseases.[52]

The use of bisphosphonates, particularly pamidronate, has been shown to be effective at reducing pain in FD.[53] Surgery is indicated in the case of persistent pain despite medical therapy, correction of deformity, pathological fracture, and transformation of the lesions into either benign (i.e., aneurysmal bone cyst) or malignant tumors.[54] Standard surgical management consists of curettage and bone grafting. Unlike the majority of bone lesions, allogeneic grafts are preferred over autogenous ones due to slower replacement rate by host bone, increasing the duration of the graft.[44] Simple curettage and bone grafting do not usually correct a marked deformity or restore the function of a limb. In these cases, osteotomies and fixed-angled internal-fixation devices are required.

CYSTIC LESIONS: UNICAMERAL BONE CYST, ANEURYSMAL BONE CYST

Unicameral bone cysts (UBCs), also known as simple bone cysts, comprise 3% of all bone tumors and affect predominantly children and adolescents, with peak incidence between ages of 3 and 14.[55] UBCs usually arise in long bones, most often in their proximal end and within the medullary canal. Although potentially occurring in any bone, the proximal humerus and proximal femur account for > 90% of cases.[56]

The majority of patients with UBCs are asymptomatic, and the diagnosis is typically reached through incidental plain radiographs. In symptomatic patients, pain is the most common complaint; mild pain may indicate a microscopic pathologic fracture, while a more abrupt course after a minor trauma can occur after an overt pathologic fracture.[57] In the latter, pain might be accompanied by swelling, erythema, and/or deformity.

Aneurysmal bone cysts (ABCs) are the second most common bone cystic lesion in children, comprising about 1% of all bone tumors. Around 75–90% of all ABCs occur in patients younger than 20 years, with a slight predilection for men.[58] Long bones and the spine are usually affected, with the femur (22%), tibia (17%), spine (15%), humerus (10%), pelvis (9%) and fibula (9%) being the most common locations.[59] Lesions are normally located in the metaphyseal region.

Seventy percent of ABCs are considered to be primary lesions, while the remaining 30% usually arise from primary tumors such as UBC, chondroblastoma, giant cell tumor (GCT), osteoblastoma, CMF, NOF, FD, or telangiectatic osteosarcoma (TOS).[60] Unlike UBCs, ABCs typically present with symptoms, the most common being pain and swelling. Patients might also present pathologic fractures.

Radiological findings

Plain radiographs are always the first imaging modality requested when suspecting a UBC. An intramedullary, lytic, and expansile lesion with cortical thinning in a long bone is the most common radiographic finding.[55] Although the cortex is thinned, cortical break and periosteal reaction are usually absent.[61] Rarely, the cortex can fracture and settle in the most dependent part of the fluid-filled cyst forming the "fallen leaf sign" (Fig. 7).

Radiographic features also allow for the classification of UBCs into active and latent lesions according to distance from the growth. UBCs are classified as active when they are within 1 cm of the physis and latent as they progress toward the diaphysis.[61] Active lesions typically have a higher risk of pathologic fracture, physeal damage, and associated consequences such as growth arrest, deformity, or limb-length inequality.[62] Active lesions are most common in

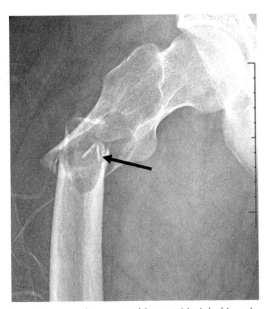

Fig. 7. Twenty-three-year-old man with right hip pain. AP radiograph of the right proximal femur demonstrates a pathologic fracture through a well-defined geographic lytic lesion in the subtrochanteric region. Note the cortical bone fragments displaced into the lesion (*arrow*), a characteristic "fallen fragment" sign of pathologic fractures in UBCs.

young patients and also show a higher rate of failure to treatment.[63]

When lesions are not easily evaluated through plain radiographs or there is a concern for bone structural integrity, we recommend performing a CT scan.[64] Three parameters have been shown to be the most accurate in predicting the risk of fracture: bone cyst index, bone cyst diameter, and minimal cortical thickness. A bone cyst index >4 for the humerus and >3.5 for the femur indicate high risk for fracture.[65] Similarly, bone cyst diameter >85% in both anteroposterior and lateral images and minimal cortical thickness < 2 mm predict a high risk of fracture.[65,66]

Classic radiographic appearance of ABCs is usually found during the stabilization phase and consists of a well-defined, expansile osteolytic lesion and possible soap-bubble appearance due to osseous septations (Fig. 8A).[67] Due to their expansive nature, lesions may elevate the periosteum but typically do not penetrate the bone cortex.[58] ABCs are typically located in the metaphyseal portion of the bone; when lesions are located in the epiphysis, physicians should suspect a different bone lesion.[68]

MRI is a valuable tool to aid diagnosis and typically shows cystic formation fluid-fluid levels

due to blood sedimentation (Fig. 8B and C). Although suggestive, this imaging pattern is not pathognomonic of ABC and may be also observed in other bone tumors such as TOC, GCT, and fracture through UBC.[58] Unlike other bone tumors, ABCs require a histological diagnosis before treatment to rule out associated malignant tumors.

Treatment

UBCs in asymptomatic patients without compromise of bone structure nor risk of further expansion are usually treated conservatively with observation. Furthermore, when patients with a UBC develop a pathologic fracture of the upper limb, we recommend nonsurgical treatment with immobilization for 4 to 6 weeks.[64]

To date, no universal definition of cyst resolution/healing has been implemented. For practical purposes, we define complete healing as >95% opacification of the cyst with cortical thickening and no pain.[64] It has been postulated that after the resolution of a pathologic fracture, spontaneous healing of the UBC may follow. However, studies show a significantly low rate of spontaneous resolution after a pathologic fracture, perhaps as low as 5%.[57]

Candidates for invasive treatment include those with symptomatic cysts, pathologic fracture, cyst expansion during observation, and cyst location in an area with a high risk of fracture. Invasive treatment is usually divided into 3 categories: injection techniques, surgical techniques, and combined techniques.

Methylprednisolone injections were the first to be used but their use has been progressively diminishing due to newer studies showing a 15%–88% recurrence rate after an average of 3 steroid injections.[69] Recently, autologous bone marrow (ABM) has been suggested as a viable alternative to steroids with a lower recurrence rate.

Classically, UBCs that fitted the criteria for surgery were treated with curettage and bone grafting. However, studies demonstrated that after this treatment modality, healing rates were between 25 and 36%, only improving slightly (37% to 50%) after a second procedure was performed.[70] Decompression techniques are a set of more recent treatment modalities with a significantly higher success rate than traditional open curettage. Canavese and colleagues[71] reported a 70% success rate with percutaneous curettage (decompression) for UBC, compared with 41% and 21% of steroid and ABM injections, respectively. More recent literature on decompressive therapy has focused

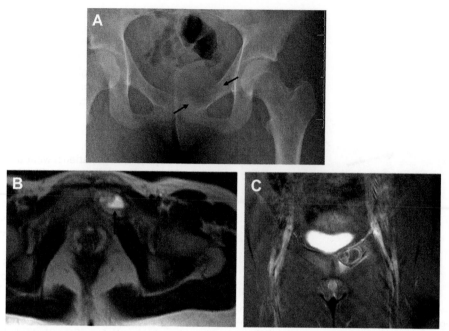

Fig. 8. Fifteen-year-old female with left pelvic pain. (A) AP radiograph demonstrates a geographic lytic lesion with sharp but nonsclerotic margins (arrows) in the left superior pubic ramus, with the erosion of the superior cortex. (B) Axial T2-weighted MRI demonstrates the characteristic fluid-fluid levels (arrow) seen in aneurysmal bone cyst, representing gravity-dependent layering of blood products. This nonspecific finding may also be seen in secondary ABC formation associated with underlying giant cell tumor of bone, chondroblastoma, or telangiectatic osteosarcoma. (C) Coronal fat-suppressed contrast-enhanced MRI demonstrates thin septal enhancement internally and peripherally but no areas of solid enhancement in this cystic neoplasm. Mild perilesional enhancement medially likely owes to stress reaction across the weakened pubic ramus.

on the use of intramedullary nails, with a healing rate > 80% at a mean follow-up of 9.8 years.[72]

Combined techniques comprise the combination of surgical techniques with biologic agents to improve treatment success. Most of the techniques include the use of intramedullary decompression followed by the injection of active compounds such as calcium sulfate pellets or 95% ethanol solution. Complete healing rates have been reported to be > 90%.[73]

Treatment of ABCs is always invasive and consists of minimally invasive and surgical treatment. Surgical treatment with curettage and bone grafting with or without adjuvant therapy is the most commonly employed treatment modality. Due to a reported recurrence of 50% after the use of simple curettage, the use of adjuvant therapy has been described in the literature.[74] In addition, Gibbs and colleagues[75] showed that curettage with a high-speed burr reduced recurrence rates independent of the graft used, reporting an overall recurrence of 12% in 34 patients treated. We recommend preoperative embolization for tumors located in highly vascularized areas to minimize intraoperative bleeding.

Most commonly used minimally invasive techniques include cryotherapy and sclerotherapy. Schreuder and colleagues[76] found a 3.7% recurrence rate in 80 patients with ABCs treated with cryotherapy and curettage. Sclerotherapy is based on the principle of cauterizing a vascular malformation which led to the development of the ABC in the first place. Among available agents, polidocanol is one of the most commonly employed, with reports of a healing rate of 97% in patients with ABCs treated with it.[77]

Although presenting the lowest rate of recurrence, en bloc resection is only used in expendable locations due to associated complications such as bleeding and growth disturbance. Patients who undergo en bloc resection often require a second reconstructive procedure due to the bone defect generated. We suggest considering this alternative when the lesion is located in bones that do not compromise the patient's functionality or for lesions that have destroyed the metaphyseal bone in periarticular areas.

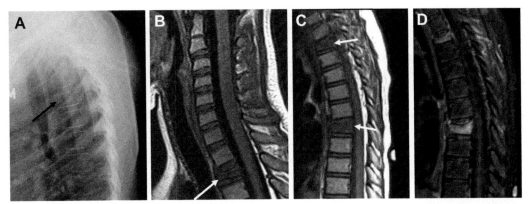

Fig. 9. Eight-year-old female with back pain. (A) Lateral radiograph of the thoracic spine demonstrates only subtle loss of anterior height in the T4 vertebral body (arrow). (B) Sagittal T1-weighted MRI of the C-spine and (C) T-spine show multiple involved vertebral bodies with compression fractures at T2 and T7 (arrows). Continued height loss may ultimately lead to vertebra plana. (D) Sagittal fat-suppressed contrast-enhanced MRI shows enhancement in the involved vertebral bodies, with biopsy eventually confirming Langerhans cell histiocytosis.

OTHER BONE TUMORS: LANGERHANS CELL HISTIOCYTOSIS

Langerhans cell histiocytosis (LCH) is a rare disease that often compromises the bone and is most common in the pediatric population. Around 50 to 90% of cases arise in patients between 1 and 15 years of age, and the reported incidence in this group is 2 to 9 cases per million.[78] LCH may compromise any organ of the body and is often divided into 2 groups depending on the extent of disease: single-system LCH and multisystem LCH. Bone is affected in 80% of patients and lesions usually occur in the vertebral bodies, long bones, and mandibles.[78] Some patients will not present symptoms at diagnosis, while others may present with pain and swelling localized in the involved area.

Other than the bone, other commonly affected organs in LCH include the skin (36%) and pituitary gland (25%).[79] Due to possible extensive compromise, when LCH is suspected, a thorough examination accompanied by complementary tests and imaging is mandatory. A bone biopsy is always necessary to reach a diagnosis.

Radiological findings
Typical radiographic features include a lytic lesion with either poorly defined borders or well-demarcated margins (Fig. 9A).[80] The lesion may or may not show reactive sclerosis and is typically located in the diaphysis or metaphysis of long bones; when found in the metaphysis, invasion of the growth plate is not common.[78] A pattern of endosteal scalloping may also be

described in long bones, giving the tumor an appearance of budding lesions. Additional features such as cortical thickening usually correlate with decreased tumor aggressiveness.[80]

It is important to differentiate LCH from other lytic lesions, such as multiple myeloma, Ewing sarcoma, and rhabdomyosarcoma. In these cases, an MRI can aid in the diagnosis of LCH through the analysis of additional parameters. Hashmi and colleagues[81] found that LCH presented less bone marrow and soft tissue edema compared to other radiographically similar tumors. In addition to help reach the diagnosis, MRI has also shown to correlate precisely with histologic grading. Lesions with high cellularity typically show high intensity on the T2 sequence, while inactive lesions demonstrate low intensity on T1 and T2 sequences (Fig. 9B–D).[82]

Treatment
Patients with LCH are typically stratified into 3 categories: isolated bone lesion (monostotic), multiple bone lesions without systemic compromise (polyostotic), and disseminated multisystem disease. For the purpose of this review, we will briefly cover the treatment of bone lesions.

The literature suggests that most lesions achieve complete or partial healing through observation alone or after a biopsy in asymptomatic monostotic disease.[83] Treatment alternatives for symptomatic patients or those with actively expanding lesions include NSAIDs, steroid injections, RT, and/or surgery. When lesions are extremely painful or are located in an anatomically difficult to reach region, low-dose radiation therapy is a good treatment alternative. Surgery is indicated when patients present neurologic deficits, usually in the setting of vertebral compromise.

Treatment of polyostotic LCH relies mainly on systemic therapy. Baptista and colleagues[84] showed how the combination of chemotherapy and steroids achieved a remission rate of 97%, while those treated with steroids alone only achieved remission in 66% of cases. Radiotherapy is often administered as an adjuvant, achieving excellent results, but patients should always be aware of the risk of side effects such as localized growth cessation and RT-associated fractures.

DISCLOSURE

The authors have nothing to disclose.

REFERENCES

1. Bergovec M, Kubat O, Smerdelj M, et al. Epidemiology of musculoskeletal tumors in a national referral orthopedic department. A study of 3482 cases. Cancer Epidemiol 2015;39(3):298–302.
2. CAFFEY J. On fibrous defects in cortical walls of growing tubular bones: their radiologic appearance, structure, prevalence, natural course, and diagnostic significance. Adv Pediatr 1955;7:13–51.
3. Lodwick GS, Wilson AJ, Farrell C, et al. Determining growth rates of focal lesions of bone from radiographs. Radiology 1980;134(3):577–83.
4. Enneking WF, Spanier SS, Goodman MA. A system for the surgical staging of musculoskeletal sarcoma. Clin Orthop Relat Res 1980;(153):106–20.
5. Ardran GM. Bone Destruction not Demonstrable by Radiography. Br J Radiol 1951;24(278):107–9.
6. Scarborough MT, Moreau G. Benign cartilage tumors. Orthop Clin North Am 1996;27(3):583–9.
7. Tong K, Liu H, Wang X, et al. Osteochondroma: Review of 431 patients from one medical institution in South China. J Bone Oncol 2017;8(1838):23–9.
8. Tepelenis K, Papathanakos G, Kitsouli A, et al. Osteochondromas: An updated review of epidemiology, pathogenesis, clinical presentation, radiological features and treatment options. Vivo (Brooklyn) 2021;35(2):681–91.
9. Frassica FJ, Frassica DA. Metastatic bone disease of the humerus. J Am Acad Orthop Surg 2003;11(4):282–8.
10. Lee EH, Shafi M, Hui JHP. Osteoid osteoma: a current review. J Pediatr Orthop 2006;26(5):695–700.
11. Tepelenis K, Skandalakis GP, Papathanakos G, et al. Osteoid osteoma: an updated review of epidemiology, pathogenesis, clinical presentation, radiological features, and treatment option. Vivo (Brooklyn) 2021;35(4):1929–38.
12. Aboulafia AJ, Kennon RE, Jelinek JS. Begnign bone tumors of childhood. J Am Acad Orthop Surg 1999;7(6):377–88.
13. Atesok KI, Alman BA, Schemitsch EH, et al. Osteoid osteoma and osteoblastoma. J Am Acad Orthop Surg 2011;19(11):678–89.
14. De Souza Diaz L, Frost HM. Osteoid osteoma–osteoblastoma. Cancer 1974;33(4):1075–81.
15. Murphey MD, Choi JJ, Kransdorf MJ, et al. Imaging of osteochondroma: variants and complications with radiologic-pathologic correlation. Radiographics 2000;20(5):1407–34.
16. Kitsoulis P, Galani V, Stefanaki K, et al. Osteochondromas: review of the clinical, radiological and pathological features. Vivo (Brooklyn) 2008;22(5):633–46.
17. Woertler K, Lindner N, Gosheger G, et al. Osteochondroma: MR imaging of tumor-related complications. Eur Radiol 2000;10(5):832–40.
18. Chai JW, Hong SH, Choi JY, et al. Radiologic diagnosis of osteoid osteoma: From simple to challenging findings. Radiographics 2010;30(3):737–49.
19. Jordan RW, Koç T, Chapman AWP, et al. Osteoid osteoma of the foot and ankle-A systematic review. Foot Ankle Surg 2015;21(4):228–34.
20. Day FN, Ruggieri C, Britton C. Recurrent osteochondroma. J Foot Ankle Surg 1998;37(2):162–4.
21. Lindquester WS, Crowley J, Hawkins CM. Percutaneous thermal ablation for treatment of osteoid osteoma: a systematic review and analysis. Skeletal Radiol 2020;49(9):1403–11.
22. Berry M, Mankin H, Gebhardt M, et al. Osteoblastoma: a 30-year study of 99 cases. J Surg Oncol 2008;98(3):179–83.
23. Dahlin DC, Ivins JC. Benign chondroblastoma. A study of 125 cases. Cancer 1972;30(2):401–13.
24. Wang J, Du Z, Yang R, et al. Analysis for clinical feature and outcome of chondroblastoma after surgical treatment: a single center experience of 92 cases. J Orthop Sci 2022;27(1):235–41.
25. Schajowicz F, Gallardo H. Epiphysial chondroblastoma of bone. A clinico-pathological study of sixty-nine cases. J Bone Joint Surg Br 1970;52(2):205–26.
26. Fink BR, Temple HT, Chiricosta FM, et al. Chondroblastoma of the foot. Foot Ankle Int 1997;18(4):236–42.
27. Rahimi A, Beabout JW, Ivins JC, et al. Chondromyxoid fibroma: a clinicopathologic study of 76 cases. Cancer 1972;30(3):726–36.
28. Wu CT, Inwards CY, O'Laughlin S, et al. Chondromyxoid fibroma of bone: a clinicopathologic review of 278 cases. Hum Pathol 1998;29(5):438–46.
29. Hakim DN, Pelly T, Kulendran M, et al. Benign tumours of the bone: a review. J Bone Oncol 2015;4(2):37–41.
30. Marco RA, Gitelis S, Brebach GT, et al. Cartilage tumors: evaluation and treatment. J Am Acad Orthop Surg 2000;8(5):292–304.

31. Maheshwari AV, Jelinek JS, Song AJ, et al. Metaphyseal and diaphyseal chondroblastomas. Skeletal Radiol 2011;40(12):1563–73.

32. De Mattos CBR, Angsanuntsukh C, Arkader A, et al. Chondroblastoma and chondromyxoid fibroma. J Am Acad Orthop Surg 2013;21(4):225–33.

33. Weatherall PT, Maale GE, Mendelsohn DB, et al. Chondroblastoma: classic and confusing appearance at MR imaging. Radiology 1994;190(2):467–74.

34. Yamaguchi T, Dorfman HD. Radiographic and histologic patterns of calcification in chondromyxoid fibroma. Skeletal Radiol 1998;27(10):559–64.

35. Murphey MD, Flemming DJ, Boyea SR, et al. From the archives of the AFIP. Enchondroma versus chondrosarcoma in the appendicular skeleton: differentiating features. Radiographics 1998;18(5):1213–37.

36. Lin PP, Thenappan A, Deavers MT, et al. Treatment and prognosis of chondroblastoma. Clin Orthop Relat Res 2005;438(438):103–9.

37. Sailhan F, Chotel F, Parot R. Chondroblastoma of bone in a pediatric population. J Bone Jt Surg - Ser A 2009;91(9):2159–68.

38. Lehner B, Witte D, Weiss S. Clinical and radiological long-term results after operative treatment of chondroblastoma. Arch Orthop Trauma Surg 2011;131(1):45–52.

39. Lersundi A, Mankin HJ, Mourikis A, et al. Chondromyxoid fibroma: a rarely encountered and puzzling tumor. Clin Orthop Relat Res 2005;439(439):171–5.

40. Andreacchio A, Alberghina F, Testa G, et al. Surgical treatment for symptomatic non-ossifying fibromas of the lower extremity with calcium sulfate grafts in skeletally immature patients. Eur J Orthop Surg Traumatol 2018;28(2):291–7.

41. Mankin HJ, Trahan CA, Fondren G, et al. Non-ossifying fibroma, fibrous cortical defect and Jaffe-Campanacci syndrome: a biologic and clinical review. Chir Organi Mov 2009;93(1):1–7.

42. Arata MA, Peterson HA, Dahlin DC. Pathological fractures through non-ossifying fibromas. J Bone Jt Surg 1981;63-A(6):980–8.

43. Vanel D, Ruggieri P, Ferrari S, et al. The incidental skeletal lesion: ignore or explore? Cancer Imaging 2009;9(SPEC. ISS. A):38–43.

44. DiCaprio MR, Enneking WF. Fibrous dysplasia: pathophysiology, evaluation, and treatment. J Bone Jt Surg - Ser A 2005;87(8):1848–64.

45. Biermann JS. Common benign lesions of bone in children and adolescents. J Pediatr Orthop 2002; 22(2):268–73.

46. Riddle ND, Bui MM. Fibrous dysplasia histopathology. Resid Short Rev 2013;137(January):134–8.

47. McCarthy EF. Fibro-osseous lesions of the maxillofacial bones. Head Neck Pathol 2013;7(1):5–10.

48. Wodajo FM. Top five lesions that do not need referral to orthopedic oncology. Orthop Clin North Am 2015;46(2):303–14.

49. Betsy M, Kupersmith LM. Springfield DS. Metaphyseal fibrous defects. J Am Acad Orthop Surg 1957; 12(2):89–95.

50. Fitzpatrick KA, Taljanovic MS, Speer DP, et al. Imaging findings of fibrous dysplasia with histopathologic and intraoperative correlation. Am J Roentgenol 2004;182(6):1389–98.

51. Shah ZK, Peh WCG, Koh WL, et al. Magnetic resonance imaging appearances of fibrous dysplasia. Br J Radiol 2005;78(936):1104–15.

52. Nakashima Y, Kotoura Y, Nagashima T, et al. Monostotic fibrous dysplasia in the femoral neck. A clinicopathologic study. Clin Orthop Relat Res 1984;191:242–8.

53. Chapurlat RD, Gensburger D, Jimenez-Andrade JM, et al. Pathophysiology and medical treatment of pain in fibrous dysplasia of bone. Orphanet J Rare Dis 2012;7(SUPPL. 1):S3.

54. Stanton RP. Surgery for fibrous dysplasia. J Bone Miner Res 2007;22(SUPPL. 2):105–9.

55. Wilkins RM. Unicameral bone cysts. J Am Acad Orthop Surg 2000;8(4):217–24.

56. Campanacci M, Capanna R, Picci P. Unicameral and aneurysmal bone cysts. Clin Orthop Relat Res 1986; 204:25–36.

57. Rosenblatt J, Koder A. Understanding unicameral and aneurysmal bone cysts. Pediatr Rev 2019; 40(2):51–9.

58. Rapp TB, Ward JP, Alaia MJ. Aneurysmal bone cyst. J Am Acad Orthop Surg 2012;20(4):233–41.

59. Cottalorda J, Kohler R, Sales De Gauzy J, et al. Epidemiology of aneurysmal bone cyst in children: A multicenter study and literature review. J Pediatr Orthop B 2004;13(6):389–94.

60. Cottalorda J, Sabah DL, Monrigal PJ, et al. Minimally invasive treatment of aneurysmal bone cysts: systematic literature review. Orthop Traumatol Surg Res 2022;103272.

61. Noordin S, Allana S, Umer M, et al. Unicameral bone cysts: current concepts. Ann Med Surg 2018;34(June):43–9.

62. Ovadia D, Ezra E, Segev E, et al. Epiphyseal involvement of simple bone cysts. J Pediatr Orthop 2003;23(2):222–9.

63. Haidar SG, Culliford DJ, Gent ED, et al. Distance from the growth plate and Its relation to the outcome of unicameral bone cyst treatment. J Child Orthop 2011;5(2):151–6.

64. Pretell-Mazzini J, Murphy RF, Kushare I, et al. Unicameral bone cysts: general characteristics and management controversies. J Am Acad Orthop Surg 2014;22(5):295–303.

65. Kaelin AJ, MacEwen GD. Unicameral bone cysts. Natural history and the risk of fracture. Int Orthop 1989;13(4):275–82.

66. Ahn JI, Park JS. Pathological fractures secondary to unicameral bone cysts. Int Orthop 1994;18(1):20–2.

67. Deventer N, Deventer N, Gosheger G, et al. Current strategies for the treatment of solitary and aneurysmal bone cysts: A review of the literature. J Bone Oncol 2021;30:100384.

68. Capanna R, Bertoni F, Bettelli G, et al. Aneurysmal bone cysts of the pelvis. Arch Orthop Trauma Surg 1986;105(5):279–84.

69. Oppenheim WL, Galleno H. Operative treatment versus steroid injection in the management of unicameral bone cysts. J Pediatr Orthop 1984;4(1):1–7.

70. Sung AD, Anderson ME, Zurakowski D, et al. Unicameral bone cyst: a retrospective study of three surgical treatments. Clin Orthop Relat Res 2008;466(10):2519–26.

71. Canavese F, Wright JG, Cole WG, et al. Unicameral bone cysts: comparison of percutaneous curettage, steroid, and autologous bone marrow injections. J Pediatr Orthop 2007;31(1):50–5.

72. Masquijo JJ, Baroni E, Miscione H. Continuous decompression with intramedullary nailing for the treatment of unicameral bone cysts. J Child Orthop 2008;2(4):279–83.

73. Hou HY, Wu K, Wang CT, et al. Treatment of unicameral bone cyst: a comparative study of selected techniques. J Bone Jt Surg - Ser A 2010;92(4):855–62.

74. Grahneis F, Klein A, Baur-Melnyk A, et al. Aneurysmal bone cyst: a review of 65 patients. J Bone Oncol 2019;18(March):1–6.

75. Gibbs CP, Hefele MC, Peabody TD, et al. Aneurysmal bone cyst of the extremities. Factors related to local recurrence after curettage with a high-speed burr. J Bone Joint Surg Am 1999;81(12):1671–8.

76. Schreuder HW, Veth RP, Pruszczynski M, et al. Aneurysmal bone cysts treated by curettage, cryotherapy and bone grafting. J Bone Joint Surg Br 1997;79(1):20–5.

77. Rastogi S, Varshney MK, Trikha V, et al. Treatment of aneurysmal bone cysts with percutaneous sclerotherapy using polidocanol. J Bone Jt Surg - Ser B 2006;88(9):1212–6.

78. DiCaprio MR, Roberts TT. Diagnosis and management of langerhans cell histiocytosis. J Am Acad Orthop Surg 2014;22(10):643–52.

79. Leung AKC, Lam JM, Leong KF. Childhood Langerhans cell histiocytosis: a disease with many faces. World J Pediatr 2019;15(6):536–45.

80. Stull MA, Kransdorf MJ, Devaney KO. Langerhans cell histiocytosis of bone. RadioGraphics 1992;12(4):801–23.

81. Hashmi MA, Haque N, Chatterjee A, et al. Langerhans cell histiocytosis of long bones: MR imaging and complete follow up study. J Cancer Res Ther 2012;8(2):286–8.

82. Moon T, Lee J, Lee I, et al. MRI and histopathologic classification of langerhans cell histiocytosis. Curr Med Imaging Rev 2009;5(1):14–8.

83. Ghanem I, Tolo VT, D'Ambra P, et al. Langerhans cell histiocytosis of bone in children and adolescents. J Pediatr Orthop 2003;23(1):124–30.

84. Baptista AM, Camargo AFF, De Camargo OP, et al. Does adjunctive chemotherapy reduce remission rates compared to cortisone alone in unifocal or multifocal histiocytosis of bone? Clin Orthop Relat Res 2012;470(3):663–9.

Hand and Wrist

Giant Cell Tumor of the Distal Radius: A Review

Matthew C. Hess, MD*, Lisa Kafchinski, MD, Erin Ransom, MD

KEYWORDS

• Giant cell tumor • Distal radius • Wrist • Allograft • Reconstruction • Arthrodesis

KEY POINTS

- Despite high recurrence rates associated with curettage and grafting, this is often the preferred initial management of giant cell tumor (GCT) of the distal radius to preserve function, as future resection of the distal radius is possible if recurrence or poor functional outcomes necessitate.
- GCT can mimic sarcomatous tumors, metastatic disease, lymphoma, and myeloma; therefore, a confirmatory biopsy is essential.
- Adjuvants after intralesional curettage, whether mechanical, thermal, or chemical, have been shown to decrease overall local recurrence rates, but no definitive difference in recurrence or superiority for a single entity has been demonstrated.
- After wide resection, no clear functional difference exists between the numerous reconstructive options.

INTRODUCTION

Background

Although relatively rare and technically a benign condition, giant cell tumor (GCT) of the distal radius presents a significant challenge in management due to its high risk of recurrence and potential loss of function. GCT of the distal radius often presents as an aggressive, lytic destruction near the highly functional wrist joint in middle-aged patients. First described in 1818 by Cooper and Travers, GCT of bone was quickly noted to be locally destructive and later found to have a neoplastic origin with metastatic potential.[1,2] Its name derives from the characteristic multinucleated, osteoclast-like giant cells seen on histopathology, which cause bone resorption.[3] However, current evidence suggests the mononuclear stromal cell is the neoplastic cell, with mutations in histone 3, H3F3A, which is now a dedicated diagnostic immunohistochemistry marker.[4,5] The osteolysis in GCT often occurs in the metaphysis and epiphysis of long bones, most often around the knee, and is very rarely multicentric except in younger patients.[6,7] The distal radius is the third most common presenting location, with GCT of bone representing approximately 20% of all biopsy-proven benign bone tumors.[8] Classically and based on recent meta-analysis, these tumors most commonly occur in patients aged 20 to 40 years and are rarely seen in adolescents or in patients with open physes.[2,9,10] Some case series suggest a slightly higher female:male ratio of patients presenting with the disease.[11,12]

Clinical Presentation

GCT of the distal radius may present late due to the non–weight-bearing nature of the wrist joint and the relatively slow-growing nature of the tumors. The most common presenting symptom is wrist pain, whether from the gradual osteolytic process or a distinct pathologic fracture.[5] Patients may also present with tenderness or swelling about the wrist joint or restricted joint motion that has been managed conservatively until a screening radiograph shows characteristic

The authors have nothing to disclose.

Department of Orthopaedic Surgery, University of Alabama-Birmingham, 1313 13th Street South, Birmingham, AL 35205, USA

* Corresponding author.

E-mail address: mattcharleshess@gmail.com

boney destruction and prompts referral. Patients are more likely to present with a pathologic fracture in one of the weight-bearing bones, most commonly the distal femur.[13] Fig. 1 shows an example of a relatively late presentation of a patient with a painful, swollen wrist for several months ultimately found to have GCT of the distal radius.

Radiographic Evaluation

Conventional radiographs very typically demonstrate a large, eccentric, meta-epiphyseal lytic lesion without matrix mineralization. The margin is varied and ranges from well-defined to poorly defined and "moth eaten" depending on the radiographic grade of the tumor. The tumor may expand the bone, elevate the periosteum, or invade the subchondral bone and articular surface. Occasionally, there is an associated soft tissue mass that is typically encapsulated by a thin rim of bone forming a so-called neocortex. GCT of the distal radius rarely involves the adjacent ulna, radiocarpal joint, or carpal bones at presentation. Isolated GCT of the distal ulna has been described and is an even more rare entity (0.45%–3.2% of all primary GCT of bone).[14] Fig. 2 demonstrates examples of characteristic radiographic findings from 2 different patients.

Radiographic Grading System

Both Enneking[15] and Campanacci[9] described staging systems for GCT of bone based on plain radiographs, which are useful for guiding management. In the Campanacci system, grade 1 lesions are very rare, constituting just 3.8% of 186 cases reviewed in a multicenter Canadian study.[7] Grade 1 lesions are well circumscribed and do not disrupt the cortex. Grade 2 lesions distort and expand the surrounding cortex but do not extend into the soft tissues. Grade 3 have an ill-defined border, disrupt the cortex, and have an associated soft tissue component. Grade 1 and 2 lesions typically are treated with intralesional curettage, whereas grade 3 lesions are more likely to require an en-bloc resection.[9]

Advanced Imaging and Timing of Biopsy

In Campannaci grade 1 or 2 lesions, it may be reasonable to obtain an intraoperative frozen pathology section to confirm the diagnosis of GCT and proceed with intralesional curettage and grafting. However, for lesions that are not classic in radiograph appearance and for higher grade lesions, advanced imaging and a core needle biopsy are indicated. There are limited guidelines for biopsy of the distal radius,[16] but when a biopsy is performed it should be done after advanced imaging so as not to disrupt the definition and characterization of the local extent of the tumor.[5] A biopsy is recommended for aggressive-appearing lesions that can mimic sarcomas. Ultrasound-guided or computed tomography (CT)-guided core needle biopsy performed by a musculoskeletal radiologist is a common method of biopsy.

A CT scan can be used to better delineate the involvement of the articular surface and subchondral bone. MRI may characterize an associated soft tissue mass. On MRI, GCT of bone is typically intermediate or low signal on T1-weighted sequences, bright on T2-weighted images, and avidly enhanced on post-gadolinium images due to the hypervascular nature.[17] Secondary aneurysmal bone cysts (ABC), which show fluid-fluid levels on MRI, occur in up to 14% of cases of GCT of bone[18] and may portend a higher recurrence rate.[19] Several pathologic processes can mimic GCT of bone and are summarized in Table 1.[17]

Histopathology

Histopathology is needed to distinguish GCT of bone from malignant or metastatic lesions. Histology exhibits multinucleated osteoclast-like giant cells that are spread evenly throughout mononuclear stromal cells that are the driving cell type in this mesenchymal tumor. The giant cells have multiple nuclei that are central and

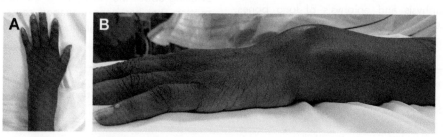

Fig. 1. (*A*) Anterior-posterior (AP) view of the left wrist of a 44-year-old woman who presented with wrist pain, swelling, and limited function. (*B*) Lateral view of the same patient's left wrist.

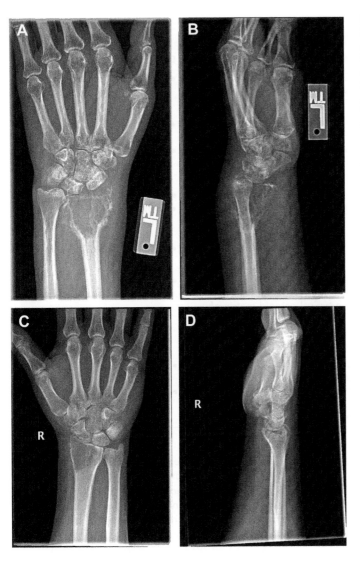

Fig. 2. (A) AP wrist radiograph. (B) Lateral wrist radiograph. (A) and (B) demonstrate an aggressive grade 3 lesion with loss of cortex and associated soft tissue component. There is involvement of the subchondral bone and collapse of the radiocarpal joint. These radiographs correspond with the patient from Fig. 1. (C): AP wrist radiograph. (D) Lateral wrist radiograph. (C) and (D) show a second patient with a less aggressive grade 2 lesion with cortical thinning but no clear extension into the soft tissue.

surrounded by ample eosinophilic cytoplasm, whereas the stromal cells show ill-defined borders and have a similar appearing central, single nuclei and scant eosinophilic cytoplasm. This fibroblastic-osteoblastic stromal cell produces types I and II collagen whose pink staining composes the background of the typical histologic slide.[5] Extensive necrosis and hemorrhage may obscure these typical features. Grossly, the tumor on intralesional resection may seem friable, soft tan-red, and hemorrhagic, as seen in Fig. 3.[21]

Metastatic Potential and Additional Workup

Further imaging workup includes screening chest imaging, such as a standard chest radiograph or a CT scan. GCT of bone has a low metastatic potential, with metastases most commonly occurring in the lung that are considered benign because they are rarely lethal.[14,22] These metastases have a low growth rate and show the same pathology as the tissue at the primary site of the tumor.[23] Differing case series suggest an approximately 2%5% occurrence among all reported GCT of bone.[24–26] In one study, metastases were detected at an average of 2 years from presentation, with approximately 50% of patients experiencing some local recurrence before or at the time of detection.[26] GCT of the distal radius historically is thought to have a higher rate of metastasis than GCT present in other common locations[24,27] but more recent case series have not observed the same trend.[26] Upper limb location may shorten

Table 1
Differential diagnosis by imaging

Diagnosis	Similar Feature	Distinguishing Feature
Primary ABC	• Cystic appearance • Meta-epiphyseal location • Fluid-fluid levels on MRI	• Primary ABC lacks soft tissue tissue component
Chondroblastoma	• Young age • Epiphyseal location • Secondary ABC formation	• Radiograph may show chondroid matrix • MRI with increased signal in surrounding soft tissue and marrow edema
Metastatic Disease • Thyroid carcinoma • Renal cell carcinoma Multiple myeloma (MM) Plasmacytoma (solitary MM)	• Lytic lesion with nonsclerotic margin	• Age typically >40 years old • Typically multiple lesions, whereas GCT is usually unicentric • Distal radius is unusual location for metastases
Osteosarcoma subtypes: • Telangiectatic • Giant cell-rich • Fibroblastic	• Lytic, aggressive lesion • Subtypes often do not have the typical osteoid matrix of conventional osteosarcoma on radiograph • Secondary ABC formation	• Need biopsy and histopathology to distinguish
Clear cell chondrosarcoma	• Lytic lesion with nonsclerotic margin near subchondral bone • Often extends into the epiphysis	• Distal radius is unusual location for chondrosarcoma • Chondroid matrix on radiographs in approximately one-third of cases[20]

the time to presentation of metastases.[22] It remains unclear why these benign lesions metastasize, but even patients with untreated pulmonary metastases, which rarely spontaneously regress, have good long-term prognosis and survival.[26,28,29] Lung nodules greater than 5 mm show higher rates of progression and warrant closer observation and consideration for treatment such as medical therapy or surgical resection.[26,29] Handling of further screening and defining the correct interval and modality for screening after presentation remains controversial. Some orthopedic oncologists will perform a chest radiograph at presentation and then no additional screening chest imaging, unless the patient presents with local recurrence or had a chest imaging abnormality on initial presentation.

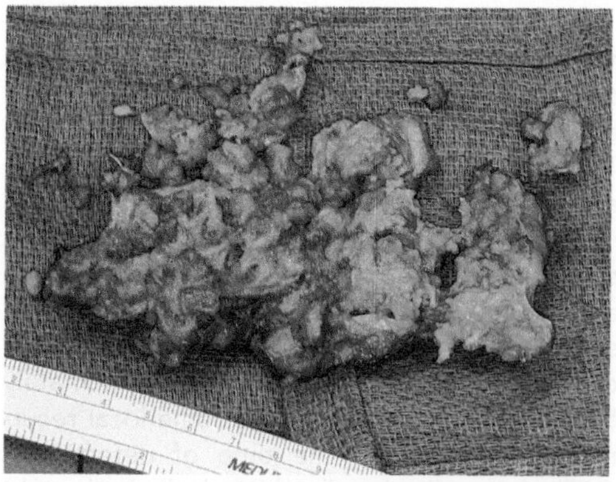

Fig. 3. The gross appearance of the aggressive grade 3 lesion seen in the same patient from Figs. 1, 2A, B, and 5. Once the thinned cortex is violated and the tumor extends into the soft tissue, it may be difficult to resect en-bloc.

Recurrence

Despite its benign categorization, GCT of bone is well known to have a relatively high risk of local recurrence regardless of the chosen surgical treatment option.[5,14] Historically, the upper extremity and the distal radius locations are reported to have a higher risk of recurrence than other sites, with 35% (17/49) of operatively treated GCT of the distal forearm showing recurrence in an early series.[30] A more recent single-center retrospective review also suggests that distal radius location contributed at least 16% to recurrence in a multivariate model.[31] The high recurrence rate in distal radius tumors is thought to often be related to inadequate excisional margins due to the close proximity to the wrist joint and an aim for preservation of function.[16,32] A recent systematic review and meta-analysis reported that, particularly in grade 3 lesions, intralesional curettage compared with en-bloc resection in the treatment of GCT of the distal radius increased the rate of local recurrence.[10] Recurrence of GCT usually occurs within 1 to 2 years but may be significantly delayed, even up to 2 decades.[30] The presence of a secondary ABC may increase recurrence rate.[19] Pathologic fracture at presentation does not increase local recurrence risk or preclude curettage as a treatment option.[33] When recurrence occurs, patients often present once more with pain and swelling in the wrist. Radiographs will show new areas of lucency around a site of prior curettage and packing as illustrated in Fig. 4. Occasionally, patients may present with new soft tissue masses around the wrist or new boney lesions. Although the rate of local recurrence is high, GCT of bone does not typically undergo sarcomatous degeneration such as seen in other benign lesions such as enchondroma or osteochondroma.[21]

DISCUSSION
Overview of Decision-Making in Management
Similar to many orthopedic oncologic conditions, there is much debate regarding optimal management amid a paucity of high-level evidence. Surgical management is the mainstay of treatment; however, medical therapies such as denosumab, which was approved for use in 2013, are continuing to spur debate over optimal treatment strategy.[4] The 2 broad categories of surgical treatment include intralesional curettage versus en-bloc resection (Table 2). Despite the absence of level 1 or 2 evidence, numerous treatment strategies exist and continue to emerge based largely on recommendations derived from case series. The known higher recurrence rate for intralesional curettage, functional demands of the wrist, and differing patient expectations make treatment selection a challenge. Shared decision-making is paramount in selecting an individualized treatment option for each patient and each presentation of GCT of the distal radius; this is highlighted by the 2 cases presented throughout this article. The first representative patient is a 44-year-old woman with already poor wrist function and significant pain in the wrist who is retired with little functional demands (see Figs. 1, 2A, B, and 3; Fig. 5). She opted to have the

tumor resected en-bloc with a subsequent wrist arthrodesis to minimize risk of reoperation and recurrence. The other patient is a 49-year-old man who plays golf multiple times a week and whose wrist function is extremely important to him (see Fig. 2C, D; Fig. 6). Knowing the risk of recurrence, he opted to try for intralesional curettage for his grade 2 lesion to have the best chance of preserving his wrist joint.

In general, when the tumor is contained within the bone (grade 1 and 2 lesions), intralesional curettage is a good option. If the tumor extends beyond bone or closely abuts the radiocarpal joint, en-bloc resection is more strongly considered.

OPERATIVE TREATMENT OPTIONS
Intralesional Curettage–Adjuvants and Grafts
Early surgical management described curettage, autograft, liquid nitrogen, resection, and allograft implants but were fraught with high complications and recurrence rates.[34,35] In the 1980s, Dr Henry Mankin's team began a treatment of curettage involving phenol and hydrogen peroxide or burring plus packing with polymethylmethacrylate (PMMA), which reduced local recurrence and complication rates.[30,36] Adjuvants, whether mechanical, thermal, or chemical, have been shown to decrease recurrence rates, but no definitive difference in recurrence or superiority has been demonstrated based on the type of adjuvant used, with no randomized comparison trials to date.[7,37–40] One must weigh the possible risks and side effects of each adjuvant when choosing which to employ. Table 3 lists the multitude of various adjuvants, and Box 1 lists the grafting options used in the literature that can be used in isolation or combination with one another.[10,38] Many investigators believe the thorough mechanical debridement with a high-speed burr and full visualization with large corticotomy of the entire tumor cavity is likely the most important factor in preventing recurrence.[40,41] In the distal radius, PMMA can mechanically support the bone cavity after curettage and help prevent joint collapse but it should not be used as a thermal adjuvant and its role in preventing recurrence is unclear.[40] Autogenous or allograft bone as well as artificial bone fillers may also be used to help support the radiocarpal joint and fill the bone cavity.[39] Plate fixation is rarely needed in the setting of intralesional curettage of the distal radius as compared with lower extremity locations but can be considered.

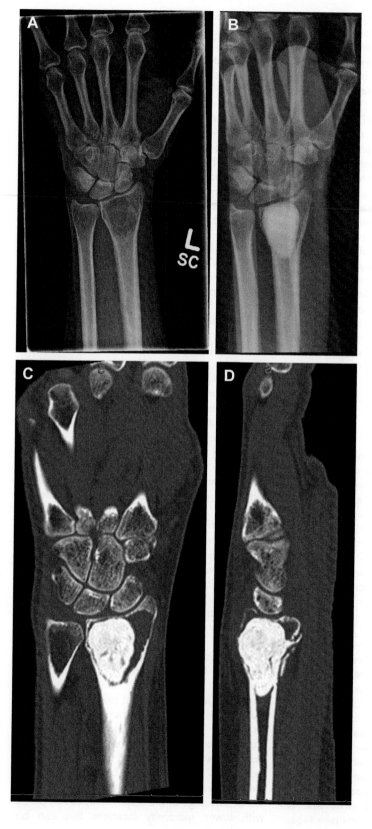

Fig. 4. A 49-year-old women who underwent curettage, irrigation with phenol and alcohol, and PMMA grafting with recurrence 3 months after surgery. (A) AP wrist radiograph at time of presentation with left wrist pain. (B) AP wrist radiograph immediately after curettage and PMMA grafting. (C) Coronal CT wrist 3 months after grafting surgery when the patient presented with increasing pain in the left wrist and screening radiograph showed concern for increasing lucency around the graft. The CT shows a progressive lucency around the radial styloid and ulnar aspect of distal radius around the PMMA graft. (D) Sagittal CT wrist 3 months after grafting surgery. The CT shows violation and fracture of the volar and dorsal cortices. The patient subsequently underwent repeat curettage and grafting.

Table 2
Summary table of treatment options

Operative: Intralesional Curettage	Operative: Wide en-Bloc Resection	Nonoperative
+/− mechanical and chemical adjuvants	+osteoarticular allograft or autograft (motion preserving)	Denosumab/bisphosphonates
+/− grafting or cementation	+biologic or prosthetic arthroplasty (motion preserving)	Embolization
+/− internal fixation	+arthrodesis	Radiation therapy

Intralesional Curettage–Recurrence and Function

Curettage, use of adjuvants, and grafting has become the mainstay of care for GCT of the distal radius, but local recurrence is arguably greater for intralesional curettage versus wide resection of the distal radius.[10,31] Debate remains regarding the best intervention to preserve function. In the most recent systematic review, the investigators conclude that intralesional curettage compared with en-bloc resection led to significantly few operative complications, lower pain scores, and improved overall functional outcomes.[10] Some investigators argue that despite the higher recurrence rate, an initial treatment with curettage is favorable because the functional outcomes of a resection plus arthrodesis after recurrence are not significantly different than those from an initial resection plus arthrodesis procedure.[32] Initial treatment with curettage remains a good option when, after shared decision-making, functional benefits outweigh the risk of recurrence[42]; this was the case for the patient highlighted in Fig. 6. Campanacci grade 3 lesions warrant further discussion with patients, as the risk of

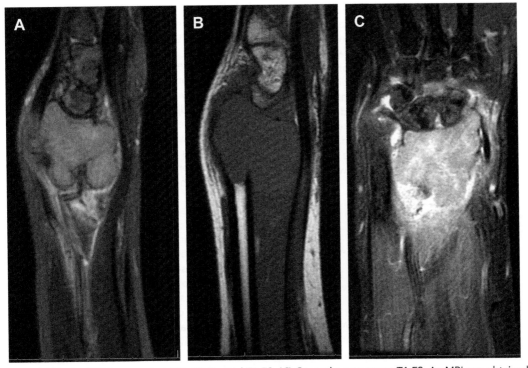

Fig. 5. (A) Sagittal T2 fat-saturated (FS). (B) Sagittal T1 FS. (C) Coronal postcontrast T1 FS. An MRI was obtained before biopsy to better characterize an aggressive appearing grade 3 lesion with a soft tissue component in preparation for a wide resection.

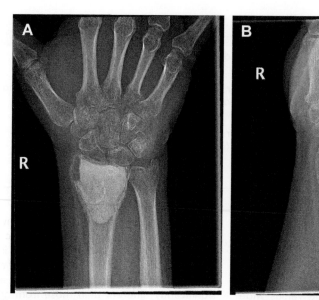

Fig. 6. The postoperative radiographs after extensive curettage with a high-speed burr, treatment with adjuvants of sterile water and hydrogen peroxide, and grafting with PMMA augmented with zoledronic acid from the same patient from **Fig. 2**C and D with a grade 2 lesion. (*A*) AP wrist radiograph. (*B*) Lateral wrist radiograph.

local recurrence with intralesional curettage is more than 5 times higher compared with en-bloc resection.[10]

En-Bloc Wide Resection

En-bloc resection is typically a good option in expendable bones such as the distal ulna, proximal and mid-fibula, and the clavicle, but for the highly function distal radius and wrist joint, it poses challenges.[5] Wide resection decreases recurrence rates in the distal radius, but the functional outcomes are worse than compared with intralesional curettage, and there are increased surgical complications regardless of the reconstruction method utilized. No option has definitively been shown to be superior to one another, and each has its own risks and benefits.[10] Depending on the specific tumor, resection can be approached volar or dorsal. Wide resection with margins following tumor principles is the goal. Because of the heterogenous nature of GCT of the distal radius, particularly Campanacci grade 3 lesions, thinning of the cortices, and associated soft tissue components, negative margins can be a challenging goal to achieve. The radiocarpal and distal radioulnar joints are often sacrificed during the resection. Contamination of the soft tissue envelope should be avoided or at least minimized with the use of adjuvants (**Table 3**) when necessary. Thorough mechanical debridement, irrigation of the soft tissues, and the use of chemical adjuvants such as hydrogen peroxide may mitigate soft tissue contamination and the risk of recurrence after an incomplete resection.

En-Bloc Resection and Osteoarticular Graft Reconstruction

Osteoarticular grafts used for reconstruction or arthrodesis can be either allogenic or autogenic and either vascularized or nonvascularized. Allografts are more commonly used but should be anatomically size-matched when possible. Allograft failure often results in definitive failure, whereas an autograft may be salvaged more easily and have higher likelihood of incorporation but at the cost of donor site morbidity and complexity of harvest.[43,44] Plates with locking screw hole options, whether placed volar, dorsal, or lateral, are used, as allografts take a

Table 3	
Adjuvant therapy options	
Mechanical/Thermal	**Chemical**
High-speed burr	Phenol
Pulsatile lavage	Hydrogen peroxide
Argon beam	Alcohol
Cryoablation/liquid nitrogen	Sterile water
Electrocautery	Bisphosphonates
	Zinc chloride
	Tincture iodine

Box 1
Grafting options

Allograft (cancellous bone)

Autograft (iliac crest, fibula)

PMMA ± antibiotics ± bisphosphonates

Calcium phosphate–based or some other artificial bone substitute filler

Combined approach

---

relatively long time to incorporate (on average 6–12 months) and it is helpful to avoid placing too many screws in the graft itself when planning a construct.[31] A plate with locking options that can also provide compression and span the entire graft is ideal for promoting integration of the allograft and preventing fracture.[45] Incorporation of a step-cut technique in graft preparation may increase chances of successful union.[46] In a case series of 27 patients with GCT of the distal radius treated with osteoarticular allograft reconstruction, the use of locking plates reduced the number of reoperations, allograft fractures, and wrist arthrodesis rates.[31] However, in this same study, the reoperation rate was 55% and conversion to arthrodesis 36% with a median time of conversion to arthrodesis at just more than 4 years. Complications and reoperation after allograft reconstruction are unfortunately common and include allograft fracture, nonunion or significantly delayed time to incorporation, development of radiocarpal osteoarthritis or instability, and infection.[43,44] Osteoarticular allograft reconstruction results in acceptable preservation of the wrist motion and moderate functional outcomes.[31,32,45,47,48] A multi-institutional retrospective study found no functional advantage of osteoarticular allograft reconstruction versus wrist arthrodesis with regard to musculoskeletal tumor society (MSTS) and Disability of the Arm, Shoulder, and Hand (DASH) scores.[44] Mean MSTS and DASH scores after osteoarticular allograft reconstruction were 21 and 34, respectively, with total wrist range of motion in flexion-extension averaging 65 degrees and pronation-supination averaging 124 degrees.[44]

En-Bloc Resection and Arthroplasty

An additional motion-sparing, but less common, treatment option includes a biological (vascularized and nonvascularized proximal fibula autografts) or nonbiological (unipolar or total wrist endoprosthesis) arthroplasty. The fibula head is used as a biological arthroplasty due to its anatomic similarities to the distal radius.[49] Both vascularized and nonvascularized grafts offer overall good functional results and motion with average MSTS and DASH scores of 25 and 13, respectively, for nonvascularized grafts and mean flexion-extension wrist motion of 101 degrees and 77.2% contralateral grip strength for vascularized grafts.[50,51] Nonvascularized grafts are less technically demanding to harvest but have higher rates of nonunion, longer time to fusion, as well as increased rate of bony resorption and collapse of the graft when compared with vascularized grafts.[49,51] Vascularized proximal fibula grafts are advantageous when osseous defects exceed 10 cm or there is significant soft tissue disruption, as they allow for an additional vascularized skin paddle.[52] Disadvantages for both include eventual degeneration of the wrist joint due to imprecise geometric congruity and risk of wrist instability. Both total and unipolar prosthetic replacements acceptably restore function and preserve motion but are very rare, often require custom implants, and have a high risk of complications.[53] Subluxation and aseptic loosening frequently occur in unipolar hemiarthroplasty, and studies of total wrist prosthesis are largely restricted to case reports.[49]

En-Bloc Resection and Arthrodesis

Reconstruction with arthrodesis after en-bloc resection of GCT of the distal radius may be either a total (spanning to metacarpal) or partial wrist (involving only the lunate, scaphoid, or both) arthrodesis and can be achieved via a number of techniques with a variety of graft options as summarized in Table 4.[49] A partial wrist fusion preserves more motion but offers a smaller surface area for fusion compared with total wrist fusion. As in other anatomic locations, the use of autograft, particularly vascularized autograft, offers a higher chance of fusion at the cost of donor site morbidity and technical harvest. Arthrodesis, using one of the options in Table 4, is the salvage procedure after failed motion-preserving surgical options such as intralesional curettage, osteoarticular graft reconstruction, or arthroplasty. Fig. 7 shows an example of a wide resection followed by total arthrodesis achieved with a bridging plate and osteoarticular allograft. The advantage of arthrodesis compared with graft reconstruction is better preservation of grip strength, prevention of wrist instability or degenerative changes especially in the context of poor soft tissue envelope, and lower risk of reoperation.[44] For

Table 4
Summary of options for wrist arthrodesis

Partial Arthrodesis	Bridging Graft for Total Arthrodesis	Ulna-Based Procedures for Total Arthrodesis
Proximal fibula autograft (± vascularized)	Osteoarticular distal radius allograft	Distal ulna centralization[55]
Tibia cortical strut allograft[56]	Proximal fibula autograft (± vascularized)	Distal ulna translocation[57]
	Iliac crest autograft (± vascularized)	Double barrel segmental ulna reconstruction combined with Sauvé-Kapandji procedure[58]

tumors that closely involve the articular surface, a recent study recommends arthrodesis over intralesional curettage for superior functional outcomes. The investigators used a free vascularized fibula graft for radiocarpal arthrodesis and reported a lower QuickDASH functional score and no differences in MSTS, Visual Analog Scale, or Patient-Rated Wrist Evaluation scores at long-term follow-up for a very small cohort of patients undergoing arthrodesis versus intralesional curettage.[54]

Further Considerations in Management After Wide Resection

Wide resection often destabilizes the wrist joint with possible excision or disruption of the wrist capsule, wrist ligaments, distal interosseous membrane, and compromise of the distal radio-ulnar joint (DRUJ).[49] Several of the ulna-based procedures for wrist arthrodesis listed in Table 4 describe methods for stabilizing the DRUJ, typically with arthrodesis of the distal ulna to the grafted distal radius via the Sauvé-Kapandji

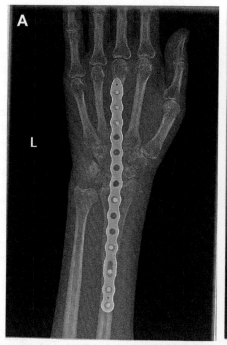
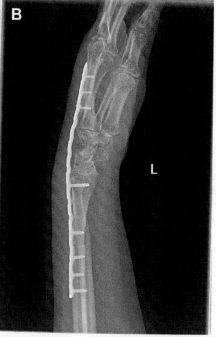

Fig. 7. (A) AP wrist radiograph. (B) Lateral wrist radiograph. Fig. 7 shows an example of a bridging distal radius osteoarticular graft fixed with a plate with locking and compression hole options for total arthrodesis for a 44-year-old woman with poor function and low demand. In this case, only the radioscaphoid and radiolunate articular surfaces were directly prepared for fusion. The plate was bent to provide slight flexion and ulnar deviation while spanning the graft, screws in the graft were minimized, and compression was provided across the graft/host bone junction.

(S-K) procedure. Combining the S-K procedure with osteoarticular allograft reconstruction after wide resection has been shown to decrease wrist instability with less degenerative wrist changes and improve function with better range of motion and grip strength.[59] If a motion-preserving reconstruction method is being used, there are few guidelines for management. If an arthrodesis or permanent ligamentous fixation method is not used, the DRUJ should be at least temporarily immobilized with a postoperative splint or with a percutaneous pinning of the intact distal ulna to the allograft distal radius.

Nonoperative Treatment

Nonoperative treatment is rarely pursued in the setting of isolated GCT of the distal radius. Modalities such as radiation and tumor embolization are often reserved for GCT of the bone in challenging-to-treat anatomic locations such as the spine and pelvis or in patients who are unable to undergo surgery secondary to medical illness.[5]

The Role of Denosumab in Giant Cell Tumor of the Distal Radius

The role of denosumab in the treatment of GCT of the distal radius stems from the receptor activator of nuclear factor kappa beta (RANK) and RANK ligand (RANKL) interaction.[60] Denosumab is a human monoclonal antibody that inhibits RANKL and may thereby have a downregulating effect on the RANK-expressing osteoclast precursor cells that ultimately contribute to bone lysis. However, denosumab does not directly target or kill the stromal neoplastic cells and is therefore not curative but mitigates its destructive effects. The US Food and Drug Administration approved its use in 2013 for skeletally mature patients with unresectable GCT of bone or advanced local disease in which surgical resection would cause morbidity.[4] Denosumab may be used to treat unresectable GCT of bone in more challenging anatomic locations than the distal radius and may also be used perioperatively. The use of denosumab before intralesional curettage may increase the risk of local recurrence, as the tumor necrosis alters the appearance and may increase the risk of incomplete curettage.[61,62] The increase in local recurrence rates has led some to recommend against its use preoperatively unless a wide resection is planned rather than curettage.[31,39] If curettage is performed, expert opinion is that it should be used for only 3 to 4 months to develop a calcific rim in the periphery but keep the tumor well defined enough for intralesional resection.[4] Common side effects include joint pain, nausea, fatigue, headache, and hypocalcemia. More serious side effects include jaw osteonecrosis as well as hypercalcemia and tumor recurrence after discontinuation of therapy. Clearly defining the optimal use, interval, and duration of treatment with denosumab in the treatment of GCT of the distal radius requires further research.[39]

SUMMARY

Despite being labeled a benign condition, GCT of the distal radius is a challenging entity to treat due to its highly functional location and often late presentation with advanced boney lysis near the wrist joint. Shared decision-making guides management for radiographically advanced lesions, as some patients may wish to undergo an intralesional curettage to preserve joint motion and function. The role of various adjuvants and graft options as well as the proper perioperative use of denosumab needs to be studied further to best understand how to mitigate recurrence and optimize functional outcomes.

CLINICS CARE POINTS

- Despite high recurrence rates associated with curettage and grafting, this is often the preferred initial management of giant cell tumor (GCT) of the distal radius to preserve function, as future resection of the distal radius is possible if recurrence or poor functional outcomes necessitate.

- GCT can mimic sarcomatous tumors, metastatic disease, lymphoma, and myeloma; therefore, a confirmatory biopsy is essential.

- Adjuvants after intralesional curettage, whether mechanical, thermal, or chemical, have been shown to decrease overall local recurrence rates, but no definitive difference in recurrence or superiority for a single entity has been demonstrated.

- After wide resection, no clear functional difference exists between the numerous reconstructive options.

DISCLOSURE

The authors have nothing to disclose.

REFERENCES

1. Cooper ATB. Surgical essays: Part I, ed 2. London, England: Cox and Son; 1818.
2. Jaffe HL. Giant-cell tumour (osteoclastoma) of bone: its pathologic delimitation and the inherent clinical implications. Ann R Coll Surg Engl 1953; 13(6):343–55.
3. Carrasco CH, Murray JA. Giant cell tumors. Orthop Clin North Am 1989;20(3):395–405.
4. Basu Mallick A, Chawla SP. Giant cell tumor of bone: an update. Curr Oncol Rep 2021;23(5):51.
5. Raskin KA, Schwab JH, Mankin HJ, et al. Giant cell tumor of bone. J Am Acad Orthop Surg 2013;21(2): 118–26.
6. Hoch B, Inwards C, Sundaram M, et al. Multicentric giant cell tumor of bone. Clinicopathologic analysis of thirty cases. J Bone Joint Surg Am 2006;88(9): 1998–2008.
7. Turcotte RE, Wunder JS, Isler MH, et al. Giant cell tumor of long bone: a Canadian Sarcoma Group study. Clin Orthop Relat Res 2002;397:248–58.
8. Baena-Ocampo Ldel C, Ramirez-Perez E, Linares-Gonzalez LM, et al. Epidemiology of bone tumors in Mexico City: retrospective clinicopathologic study of 566 patients at a referral institution. Ann Diagn Pathol 2009;13(1):16–21.
9. Campanacci M, Baldini N, Boriani S, et al. Giant-cell tumor of bone. J Bone Joint Surg Am 1987;69(1):106–14.
10. Koucheki R, Gazendam A, Perera J, et al. Management of giant cell tumors of the distal radius: a systematic review and meta-analysis. Eur J Orthop Surg Traumatol 2022. https://doi.org/10.1007/s00590-022-03252-9.
11. Vander Griend RA, Funderburk CH. The treatment of giant-cell tumors of the distal part of the radius. J Bone Joint Surg Am 1993;75(6):899–908.
12. Cheng CY, Shih HN, Hsu KY, et al. Treatment of giant cell tumor of the distal radius. Clin Orthop Relat Res 2001;383:221–8.
13. Eckardt JJ, Grogan TJ. Giant cell tumor of bone. Clin Orthop Relat Res 1986;204:45–58.
14. Goldenberg RR, Campbell CJ, Bonfiglio M. Giant-cell tumor of bone. An analysis of two hundred and eighteen cases. J Bone Joint Surg Am 1970; 52(4):619–64.
15. Enneking WF. A system of staging musculoskeletal neoplasms. Clin Orthop Relat Res 1986;204:9–24.
16. Athanasian EA. Aneurysmal bone cyst and giant cell tumor of bone of the hand and distal radius. Hand Clin 2004;20(3):269–81, vi.
17. Chakarun CJ, Forrester DM, Gottsegen CJ, et al. Giant cell tumor of bone: review, mimics, and new developments in treatment. Radiographics 2013;33(1):197–211.
18. Murphey MD, Nomikos GC, Flemming DJ, et al. From the archives of AFIP. Imaging of giant cell tumor and giant cell reparative granuloma of bone: radiologic-pathologic correlation. Radiographics 2001;21(5):1283–309.
19. Liu H, Liu D, Jiang X, et al. Aneurysmal bone cyst secondary to giant cell tumor of the extremities: a case series of 30 patients. Am J Transl Res 2022; 14(5):3198–206.
20. Collins MS, Koyama T, Swee RG, et al. Clear cell chondrosarcoma: radiographic, computed tomographic, and magnetic resonance findings in 34 patients with pathologic correlation. Skeletal Radiol 2003;32(12):687–94.
21. Organization WH. WHO classification of tumours: soft tissue and bone tumours. 5th edition. Lyon, France: International Agency for Research on Cancer; 2020.
22. Yang Y, Huang Z, Niu X, et al. Clinical characteristics and risk factors analysis of lung metastasis of benign giant cell tumor of bone. J Bone Oncol 2017;7:23–8.
23. Katz E, Nyska M, Okon E, et al. Growth rate analysis of lung metastases from histologically benign giant cell tumor of bone. Cancer 1987;59(10):1831–6.
24. Rock MG, Pritchard DJ, Unni KK. Metastases from histologically benign giant-cell tumor of bone. J Bone Joint Surg Am 1984;66(2):269–74.
25. Tubbs WS, Brown LR, Beabout JW, et al. Benign giant-cell tumor of bone with pulmonary metastases: clinical findings and radiologic appearance of metastases in 13 cases. AJR Am J Roentgenol 1992;158(2):331–4.
26. Viswanathan S, Jambhekar NA. Metastatic giant cell tumor of bone: are there associated factors and best treatment modalities? Clin Orthop Relat Res 2010;468(3):827–33.
27. Peimer CA, Schiller AL, Mankin HJ, et al. Multicentric giant-cell tumor of bone. J Bone Joint Surg Am 1980;62(4):652–6.
28. Cheng JC, Johnston JO. Giant cell tumor of bone. Prognosis and treatment of pulmonary metastases. Clin Orthop Relat Res 1997;338:205–14.
29. Tsukamoto S, Ciani G, Mavrogenis AF, et al. Outcome of lung metastases due to bone giant cell tumor initially managed with observation. J Orthop Surg Res 2020;15(1):510.
30. Harness NG, Mankin HJ. Giant-cell tumor of the distal forearm. J Hand Surg Am 2004;29(2):188–93.
31. Lans J, Oflazoglu K, Lee H, et al. Giant cell tumors of the upper extremity: predictors of recurrence. J Hand Surg Am 2020;45(8):738–45.
32. Wysocki RW, Soni E, Virkus WW, et al. Is intralesional treatment of giant cell tumor of the distal radius comparable to resection with respect to local control and functional outcome? Clin Orthop Relat Res 2015;473(2):706–15.
33. Salunke AA, Shah J, Gupta N, et al. Pathologic fracture in osteosarcoma: association with poorer overall survival. Eur J Surg Oncol 2016;42(6):889–90.

34. Sheth DS, Healey JH, Sobel M, et al. Giant cell tumor of the distal radius. J Hand Surg Am 1995; 20(3):432–40.

35. Campanacci M. Bone and soft tissue tumors: giant cell tumor. 2nd edition. Vienna, Austria: Springer Verlag; 1999.

36. O'Donnell RJ, Springfield DS, Motwani HK, et al. Recurrence of giant-cell tumors of the long bones after curettage and packing with cement. J Bone Joint Surg Am 1994;76(12):1827–33.

37. Kivioja AH, Blomqvist C, Hietaniemi K, et al. Cement is recommended in intralesional surgery of giant cell tumors: a Scandinavian Sarcoma Group study of 294 patients followed for a median time of 5 years. Acta Orthop 2008;79(1):86–93.

38. Errani C, Tsukamoto S, Ciani G, et al. Present day controversies and consensus in curettage for giant cell tumor of bone. J Clin Orthop Trauma 2019; 10(6):1015–20.

39. Nagano A, Urakawa H, Tanaka K, et al. Current management of giant-cell tumor of bone in the denosumab era. Jpn J Clin Oncol 2022;52(5):411–6.

40. Bickels J, Campanacci DA. Local Adjuvant Substances following curettage of bone tumors. J Bone Joint Surg Am 2020;102(2):164–74.

41. Gundavda MK, Agarwal MG. Extended curettage for giant cell tumors of bone: a surgeon's view. JBJS Essent Surg Tech 2021;11(3). https://doi.org/ 10.2106/JBJS.ST.20.00040.

42. Pazionis TJ, Alradwan H, Deheshi BM, et al. A systematic review and meta-analysis of En-Bloc vs intralesional resection for giant cell tumor of bone of the distal radius. Open Orthop J 2013;7: 103–8.

43. Bus MP, van de Sande MA, Taminiau AH, et al. Is there still a role for osteoarticular allograft reconstruction in musculoskeletal tumour surgery? a long-term follow-up study of 38 patients and systematic review of the literature. Bone Joint J 2017;99-B(4):522–30.

44. Bianchi G, Sambri A, Marini E, et al. Wrist arthrodesis and osteoarticular reconstruction in giant cell tumor of the distal radius. J Hand Surg Am 2020; 45(9):882 e1–6.

45. Duan H, Zhang B, Yang HS, et al. Functional outcome of en bloc resection and osteoarticular allograft reconstruction with locking compression plate for giant cell tumor of the distal radius. J Orthop Sci 2013;18(4):599–604.

46. Luchetti TJ, Wysocki RW, Cohen MS. Distal radius allograft reconstruction utilizing a step-cut technique after En bloc tumor resection. Hand (N Y) 2019;14(4):530–3.

47. Bianchi G, Donati D, Staals EL, et al. Osteoarticular allograft reconstruction of the distal radius after bone tumour resection. J Hand Surg Br 2005; 30(4):369–73.

48. Rabitsch K, Maurer-Ertl W, Pirker-Fruhauf U, et al. Reconstruction of the distal radius following tumour resection using an osteoarticular allograft. Sarcoma 2013;2013:318767.

49. Liu W, Wang B, Zhang S, et al. Wrist reconstruction after En bloc resection of bone tumors of the distal radius. Orthop Surg 2021;13(2):376–83. https://doi. org/10.1111/os.12737.

50. Qi DW, Wang P, Ye ZM, et al. Clinical and radiographic results of reconstruction with fibular autograft for distal radius giant cell tumor. Orthop Surg 2016;8(2):196–204.

51. Yang YF, Wang JW, Huang P, et al. Distal radius reconstruction with vascularized proximal fibular autograft after en-bloc resection of recurrent giant cell tumor. BMC Musculoskelet Disord 2016;17(1): 346.

52. Clarkson PW, Sandford K, Phillips AE, et al. Functional results following vascularized versus nonvascularized bone grafts for wrist arthrodesis following excision of giant cell tumors. J Hand Surg Am 2013;38(5):935–940 e1.

53. Wang B, Wu Q, Liu J, et al. What are the functional results, complications, and outcomes of using a custom unipolar wrist hemiarthroplasty for treatment of grade III giant cell tumors of the distal radius? Clin Orthop Relat Res 2016;474(12):2583–90.

54. Kuruoglu D, Rizzo M, Rose PS, et al. Treatment of giant cell tumors of the distal radius: A long-term patient-reported outcomes study. J Surg Oncol 2022. https://doi.org/10.1002/jso.26967.

55. Bhagat S, Bansal M, Jandhyala R, et al. Wide excision and ulno-carpal arthrodesis for primary aggressive and recurrent giant cell tumours. Int Orthop 2008;32(6):741–5.

56. van de Sande MA, van Geldorp NH, Dijkstra PD, et al. Surgical technique: Tibia cortical strut autograft interposition arthrodesis after distal radius resection. Clin Orthop Relat Res 2013;471(3): 803–13.

57. Chobpenthai T, Thanindratarn P, Phorkhar T, et al. The reconstruction after en-bloc resection of giant cell tumors at the distal radius: A systematic review and meta-analysis of the ulnar transposition reconstruction technique. Surg Oncol 2020;34:147–53.

58. Zhang W, Zhong J, Li D, et al. Functional outcome of en bloc resection of a giant cell tumour of the distal radius and arthrodesis of the wrist and distal ulna using an ipsilateral double barrel segmental ulna bone graft combined with a modified Sauve-Kapandji procedure. J Hand Surg Eur 2017;42(4): 377–81.

59. Li J, Jiao Y, Guo Z, et al. Comparison of osteoarticular allograft reconstruction with and without the Sauve-Kapandji procedure following tumour

resection in distal radius. J Plast Reconstr Aesthet Surg 2015;68(7):995–1002.

60. Huang L, Xu J, Wood DJ, et al. Gene expression of osteoprotegerin ligand, osteoprotegerin, and receptor activator of NF-kappaB in giant cell tumor of bone: possible involvement in tumor cell-induced osteoclast-like cell formation. Am J Pathol 2000;156(3):761–7.

61. Traub F, Singh J, Dickson BC, et al. Efficacy of denosumab in joint preservation for patients with giant cell tumour of the bone. Eur J Cancer 2016; 59:1–12.

62. Errani C, Tsukamoto S, Leone G, et al. Denosumab may increase the risk of local recurrence in patients with giant-cell tumor of bone treated with curettage. J Bone Joint Surg Am 2018;100(6):496–504.

Shoulder and Elbow

Management of Proximal Humeral Oncologic Lesions

Alexandra M. Arguello, MD, Matthew T. Houdek, MD, Jonathan D. Barlow, MD*

KEYWORDS

- Proximal humerus • Orthopedic oncology • Reconstruction • Sarcoma • Upper extremity

---

KEY POINTS

- The proximal humerus is the most common location for primary tumors and metastases in the upper extremity.
- There are a wide variety of possible surgical techniques for both metastatic lesions of the proximal humerus and primary tumors requiring negative margins, without a clear "gold standard" reconstructive technique.
- Reverse total shoulder arthroplasty with an endoprosthesis for patients with poor bone quality, and need for radiotherapy and lower functional demand and allograft-prosthesis composite for patients who are younger and higher functional demand show promising outcomes and decreased rates of instability compared with hemiarthroplasty.

INTRODUCTION/BACKGROUND/PREVALENCE

Oncologic lesions of the proximal humerus account for a broad range of pathologies including primary sarcomas such as osteosarcoma, chondrosarcoma, and Ewing sarcoma, benign lesions including osteochondroma, enchondroma, unicameral and aneurysmal bone cysts, and giant cell tumor of bone, metastatic disease, and myeloma.[1,2] Twenty percent of patients with metastatic cancer to the bone have disease in the upper extremity, with the humerus being the second most common site in the appendicular skeleton and the third most common site overall for bony metastasis.[3–8]

It is important to understand the functional anatomy of the shoulder before discussing surgical options for reconstruction after resection for tumor. The head of the humerus and the relatively flat glenoid articulate to form the shoulder joint, which is the most mobile joint in the body.[9] There are numerous static and dynamic stabilizers including the labrum, glenohumeral ligaments, capsule, rotator cuff muscles, and deltoid that prevent subluxation or dislocation of the shoulder joint while allowing for a broad range of motion. Depending on the planned resection margins, loss of stabilizing structures without appropriate reconstruction can ultimately result in an unstable and nonfunctional shoulder. The purpose of this review is to provide an overview of the evaluation of patients presenting with an oncologic lesion of the proximal humerus, discuss the management of these lesions (including surgical and adjuvant treatments), and provide an updated summary of outcomes of the various treatment options.

PATIENT EVALUATION OVERVIEW

Proximal humerus lesions have a vast differential diagnosis ranging from benign and indolent to malignant and aggressive. The age of the patient can generally help to focus on the most likely differential diagnosis. A detailed history and physical examination should assess onset, duration, signs, and symptoms including pain, diminished range of motion or function, neurovascular compromise, and rate of progression of symptoms. The past medical history and current state of health are also important for consideration of prognosis and the type of reconstructive surgery the patient may be able

---

Department of Orthopedic Surgery, Mayo Clinic, 200 First Street Southwest, Rochester, MN 55905, USA
* Corresponding author.
E-mail address: Barlow.jonathan@mayo.edu

Orthop Clin N Am 54 (2023) 89–100
https://doi.org/10.1016/j.ocl.2022.08.008
0030-5898/23/© 2022 Elsevier Inc. All rights reserved.

to tolerate. Plain radiographs of the entire humerus are the preliminary imaging modality. For some, the lesion may be discovered incidentally. Characteristics of a benign lesion of the proximal humerus include those that are well circumscribed, without cortical breech, a narrow transition zone, or have features specific to the most common benign lesions.[10] Potentially malignant lesions can cause cortical disruption, periosteal reaction, have a soft tissue component, and have a broad transition zone where it is difficult to visualize any clearly defined margin.[11] In general, any lesions concerning for potential sarcoma should be referred to a comprehensive sarcoma center before consideration of a biopsy.

The Rougraff criteria are used for skeletal metastases of unknown origin.[12] In addition to the detailed history and physical examination, this includes a series of laboratories (complete blood count, comprehensive metabolic panel, erythrocyte sedimentation rate, C-reactive protein, alkaline phosphatase, serum and urine protein electrophoresis) and imaging (CT of the chest, abdomen and pelvis). The original paper noted that additional tests could be ordered if the history and physical give clues toward a specific possible primary tumor; however, the use of this workup strategy was able to determine the primary site in 85% of patients.[12] In patients who present with an indeterminant solitary bone tumor, it is important to obtain a biopsy before any operative intervention, even in the setting of a previous malignancy.

The utilization of advanced imaging for surgical planning has transformed the way orthopedic oncologists and shoulder specialists prepare for these difficult cases.[13] Computed tomography (CT) is most useful for evaluation for periosteal disruption and mineralization of the tumor, and for the reconstruction it can be used for preoperative planning purposes.[14] MRI is useful for planning the surgical resection margins and understanding proximity of the margin to nearby critical structures such as the brachial vessels. If there is a particularly aggressive tumor with a large soft tissue component that would require resection of the critical neurovascular structures and render the arm nonfunctional, this could be a contraindication to proceeding with limb-sparing surgery and an amputation may need to be discussed.[15,16]

SURGICAL/INTERVENTIONAL TREATMENT OPTIONS

Intramedullary Nail

For patients with metaphyseal lesions of the proximal humerus, there are several surgical

techniques. Lytic lesions of the proximal humerus in an older age group are most commonly metastases, myeloma or lymphoma that can be amenable to intramedullary (IM) nail fixation.[17] In patients who have widely metastatic disease, an IM nail is one such option for fixation. IM nails are typically used for prophylactic stabilization of an impending fracture or for fixation of a pathologic fracture. These patients will classically present with limited function secondary to pain with use of the arm, and this plays a substantial role in quality of life for patients with metastatic cancer, especially when the dominant arm is affected.[7,18] Using Mirels criteria, patients with upper extremity lesions will get one point for location, so the decision to proceed with prophylactic fixation depends on the severity of pain, character of the lesion (lytic, mixed, or blastic) and the size of the lesion relative to the diameter of the humerus.[19] Evans and colleagues[20] performed a validation study for using Mirels in metastatic lesions in the humerus and found that seven or greater is the optimal score for identifying impending pathologic fracture for this population. Patient selection has been shown to be critically important for outcomes with this treatment option including pathology, prognosis/life expectancy, inability to withstand a more aggressive or open surgical procedure, bone quality, and patient goals of care.[5,18,21] Of note, in patients with a life expectancy of less than 3 months, non-operative management is commonly recommended for these patients.[22] In general, the use of IM nails requires that there is adequate proximal bone stock to allow for placement of multiple proximal screws into the humeral head and distal interlock screws, as well as a preserved glenohumeral joint to allow for range of motion of the shoulder[23] (**Fig. 1**).

In terms of technique, Alvi and Damron retrospectively reviewed 96 patients to weigh the benefits of protection of the entire humerus or femur such as avoiding reoperation for tumor progression with the risks of the procedure including sequelae of emboli.[17] The rate of complications that could potentially have stemmed from an embolic phenomenon was 13%; however, most were mild and quickly self-resolved. They found that 12% of the patients had some form of tumor progression, and 6% of the nails failed requiring revision surgery. Although this study was not specific to humeri, they concluded that the risks do not outweigh the benefits for protecting the entire long bone. This continues to be the treatment at many institutions. Outcomes are generally satisfactory with this procedure, with one study reporting 97% of

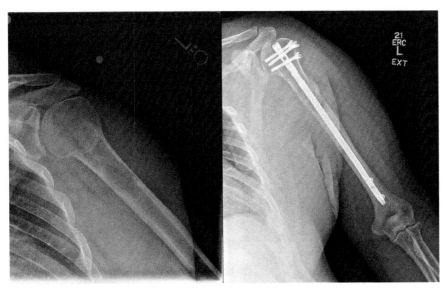

Fig. 1. 40-year-old man with a lytic lesion of the proximal humerus, biopsy confirmed multiple myeloma. Preoperative X-ray showing lytic lesion with ill-defined margins. Postoperative film of humeral nail in place.

patients having complete resolution of their arm pain after placement of an IM nail for impending fracture.[23] IM nails can fail and require subsequent surgery for a number of reasons progression or propagation of the tumor, nonunion and persistent pain, fracture of the nail itself, and infection.[21] A recent study evaluated risk factors for tumor progression and found only renal cell carcinoma primary and age to be risk factors for failure.[5] For this reason, some may choose to pursue a different surgical technique for renal cell carcinoma metastases, for example, using an endoprosthesis for those patients.[24] Cementation can also be used to fill the defect and augment the rigidity of the construct.[23] Most patients undergo some form of perioperative radiation when they have a nail placed for prophylactic purposes and a tumor sensitive to radiation.[25] In certain cases of oligometastatic disease (renal cell carcinoma), wide resection is performed rather than nailing.

Open Reduction and Internal Fixation with Locking Plate and Cementation

Open reduction and internal fixation (ORIF) with a locking plate and cementation allows for a more stable construct immediately following the procedure, allowing for the patient to weight bearing as tolerated through the arm in the immediate postoperative period.[26,27] This can be used for any lesion location in the humerus. For this technique, intralesional resection using curettes and a burr is commonly performed to minimize disease burden and decrease the risk for tumor progression.[26] Polymethylmethacrylate cement is used to

fill the defect from the tumor to provide further stability and possibly offer improved pain control.[27,28] Multiple plating methods have been described but generally one versus two plates will be used for fixation.[29] Weiss and colleagues retrospectively reviewed the 63 patients that received this fixation method for humerus lesions and found a 22% complication rate, most commonly revision for progression of disease. In the authors practice, we prefer plate fixation and cement for all lesions of the humerus (Fig. 2).

Free Vascularized Fibula

Vascularized fibular grafts can enable limb salvage by enabling reconstruction of segmental defects, or to enable fusion in the setting of substantial bony resection. This is typically completed after wide resection of primary or (rarely) metastatic disease.[30] Fuchs and colleagues[31] noted in 2005 that although endoprostheses were becoming more commonly used around that time, a shoulder arthrodesis was a reasonable procedure for some patients based on their prognosis and physical demands for the shoulder. Vascularized fibulae can be used in shoulder arthrodesis after proximal humerus tumor resection to improve the rate of fusion. The position in which patients were fused by this group was in 30° to 50° of internal rotation, 15° to 30° of abduction, and 15° to 30° of forward flexion. At mean follow-up of 11 years, patients were doing well in terms of pain control and mild disability; however, the complication rate for this procedure was 43%. Bilgin and colleagues[32] described a similar arthrodesis

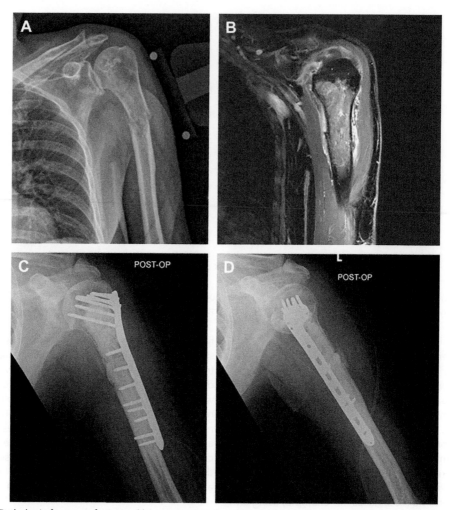

Fig. 2. Pathologic fracture of proximal humerus secondary to multiple myeloma in a 75-year-old patient. Preoperative (A) AP X-ray and (B) coronal MRI showing pathologic fracture and underlying pathology. Postoperative (C) external rotation and (D) internal rotation X-rays of the cement/plate fixation construct.

technique for a cohort of nine patients, and overall, there were reportedly good outcomes for these patients despite a 22% complication rate. In addition to restoring bone stock in the setting of shoulder arthrodesis, vascularized fibulae may be used to reconstruct diaphyseal or metaphyseal bony defects after resection or used in the setting of a nonunion.[33,34] This can be done in combination with allograft bone for additional early strength (Capanna technique).[35] The authors prefer this technique for wide, extraarticular resections, particularly in younger, higher demand patients (Figs. 3).

Osteoarticular Allografts

Osteoarticular allografting is another technique that is less commonly used but involves resection of the proximal humerus tumor and replacement with a proximal humerus allograft and fixation with a plate and screw construct with or without cement augmentation. The allograft articulates with the native glenoid and allows for a soft-tissue repair between the host and allograft tendons. DeGroot and colleagues[36] used a cemented osteoarticular allograft in their series of 31 patients requiring the procedure after resection of an aggressive proximal humerus lesion. Incidence of instability has been reported to be anywhere from 7% to 55%.[36–38] In addition, there are reports of expeditious wear of the articular cartilage, necessitating revision surgeries. Jamshidi and colleagues compared cemented and uncemented osteoarticular allografts fixed with anteromedial plating and found that the complication rate was significantly lower in the

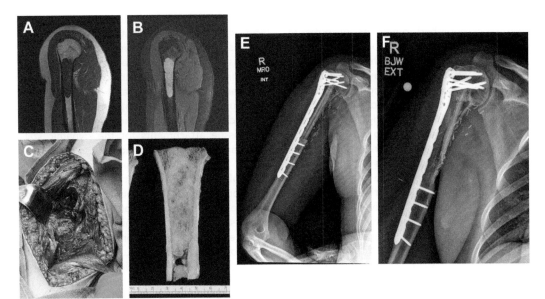

Fig. 3. Extraarticular, metaphyseal chondrosarcoma in a 20-year-old patient. (A) T1- and (B) T2-weighted preoperative MRI showing atypical cartilaginous tumor. Intraoperative photos of surgical site s/p resection (C) and (D) resected specimen. (E) Structural allograft combined with free vascularized fibular flap for reconstruction (Capanna Technique)—2 months postop and (F) 14 months postop, showing incorporation of the autograft.

cemented allografts (15% in cemented vs 80% in uncemented). The complications noted in this study included fracture, osteolysis/resorption, infection, and nonunion. The authors currently have limited indications for osteoarticular allograft use.

Arthroplasty

Henderson and colleagues[39] evaluated endoprostheses for tumor in all bones, 16% of which were proximal humerus endoprostheses. They devised a classification system for standardizing the way endoprosthetic failure is categorized. They found that the two broad categories were mechanical failure and non-mechanical failure. The three types of mechanical failure are soft tissue failure (type 1) and aseptic loosening of the implant (type 2), and structural failure or an issue with the bone quality, fracture, implant (type 3). The two nonmechanical failure mechanisms are infection (type 4) and progression of tumor (type 5). This characterization of failure types is now used throughout the literature.

Endoprosthesis

One option for reconstruction of proximal humeral lesions, particularly those that involve the joint, is an endoprosthesis. The benefit of these endoprostheses with modular components is that they allow for a prosthesis to be built up to fill in the defect in an individualized manner[13] (Fig. 5). If the glenoid cartilage is in good

condition, and the rotator cuff can be salvage, a hemiarthroplasty can be performed for proximal humerus oncologic lesions; however, the rate of complications with these implants is high, even with an adequate rotator cuff to allow for soft-tissue repair.[40–42] Without a superior soft tissue envelope, the prosthesis can migrate and impinge upon the undersurface of the acromion (or even subcutaneous) which causes both pain and decreased range of motion/function of the shoulder joint.

Reverse shoulder arthroplasty (RSA) has become the preferred means of endoprosthetic reconstruction (Fig. 4).[43,44] This technique works well in the setting of tumor because the resection margins may include some or all of the rotator cuff, which are not necessary for stability of this implant.[45] Grosel and colleagues[46] describe their endoprosthetic RSA technique and note that they increase the size of the glenosphere for all oncologic reconstructive reverse shoulders. This allows for increased stability of the construct and a lower likelihood of dislocation, which is an area of concern after a large soft tissue resection. Of note, an intact and functional deltoid has been thought to be necessary for this implant, particularly to ensure stability in the absence of other soft tissue attachments.[47] If the deltoid has been denervated by sacrifice of the axillary nerve or resection of a significant portion of muscle must be done, classic teaching is the technique will not provide the patient with an optimal functional outcome. Elhassan and colleagues[48] published outcomes of patients who underwent pectoralis flap reconstruction of the deltoid. Those patients had a mean forward elevation of 83°, which may be acceptable for some patients when weighing the remaining risks and benefits of this procedure. Cemented stems can be used in the setting of insufficient bone stock and in patients who will need postoperative radiation.[46] In addition, when the indication for endoprosthesis is a pathologic fracture, cementation should be performed.[24]

Constrained prostheses are those that use a "fixed fulcrum" and aim to solve the problem of superior migration especially in the setting of large tumor dissections.[42] Indication for the use of this in one study was soft tissue derangements that could lead to an unstable shoulder including absence of the deltoid, axillary nerve, deltoid insertion, rotator cuff, or surrounding soft tissues.[49] One such articulation is called the Bayley–Walker articulation. In comparing hemiarthroplasty to a constrained RSA, multiple studies reflect that there are significant complications associated with the constrained implant including 26% rate of failure of the constrained mechanism in one cohort and incidence of revision surgery of 18% in another study.[42,49]

As described above, is not uncommon for the soft tissue attachments for the dynamic stabilizers and muscles of the shoulder to be included within the resection margin. To maximize function of the shoulder joint after placement of endoprostheses in the shoulder, synthetic mesh has been used as a scaffold for attachment of soft tissue structures.[50] This mesh circumferentially encompasses the prosthesis and allows for those soft tissue structures to more reliably scar into an optimal location for restoration of function. Although there was some debate regarding the utility of mesh based on early data,[51–53] Tang and colleagues[54] reported

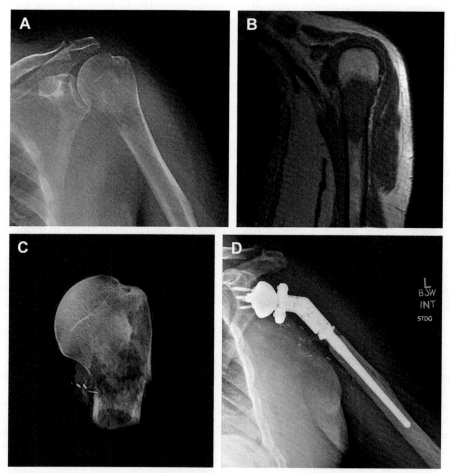

Fig. 4. 65-year-old patient with proximal humerus metastasis (renal cell carcinoma). (A) Plain film X-ray and (B) coronal T1 MRI image showing large intramedullary lesion within the proximal humeral metadiaphysis. (C) Resected surgical specimen (X-ray). (D) Endoprosthesis reconstruction of the proximal humerus.

higher functional patient reported outcome scores as well as objective range of motion in patients who had a synthetic mesh placed compared with patients without a mesh. Patients reported improved activities of daily living scores in 70% of the categories including reaching a shelf, work, and putting on a coat.

Allograft prosthetic composites

An allograft prosthetic composite (APC) involves placing a humeral arthroplasty (hemiarthroplasty or reverse total shoulder arthroplasty) into a humeral allograft that can be cut precisely to replace the defect after resection of a tumor, and subsequently fixed to the patient's remaining distal bone typically with a plate and screws.[55] A major advantage of APC in the proximal humerus is that the humeral allograft specimens may have rotator cuff attachments which allow repair of the native tendons to allograft.[24] Sanchez-Sotelo and colleagues[56] published their technique for APC with RSA in the setting of proximal humerus resection for large defects including malignancy. Utilization of an APC can be considered for younger patients with higher functional demand and long resections with minimal distal bone available for stem fixation of a megaprosthesis. A benefit of this surgical option is the ability to preserve and repair the native rotator cuff and soft tissues to the APC. In addition, the ability to measure the resected specimen and replace what has been resected with the allograft allows for the humeral length to be precisely restored and the deltoid to be adequately tensioned, resulting in improved functional outcomes and stability.[57,58] The outcomes for APCs for proximal humerus tumors are quite variable, with one systematic review of ten small studies reporting MSTS scores from 57% to 91%.[59] In addition, the rate of complications reported in the systematic review varied between 19% and 79%. A comparative study of 83 patients found that the functional outcomes after a reverse arthroplasty are improved compared with a hemiarthroplasty for intraarticular proximal humerus tumors.[24] The authors prefer APC reconstruction in young patients, and particularly in patients with resection levels distal to the deltoid attachment (see Fig. 5).

Patient specific instrumentation

Modern technology currently allows for the creation of patient-specific instrumentation including guides and protheses.[8,60] At a mean follow-up of 24 months, Hu and colleagues found that there were no hardware complications in this cohort of seven patients, including scapular notching, loosening, or dislocation and they had excellent range of motion at final follow-up. Logistical issues and cost of personalized implants will likely prevent this technology from becoming a standard treatment in the near future.

COMBINATION THERAPIES

For lesions that are appropriately treated with intralesional excision, the use of local adjuvants decreases the risk of recurrence.[61] Although the process of curettage functions to remove

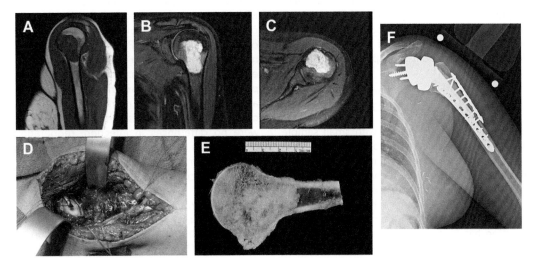

Fig. 5. 35-year-old woman with proximal humerus chondrosarcoma. (A) T1 sagittal oblique, (B) T2 coronal oblique and (C) T2 axial oblique showing indeterminate lesion eventually biopsy proven chondrosarcoma. (D) Surgical field after specimen resection and (E) Resected specimen. (F) Postoperative film demonstrating APC reverse shoulder arthroplasty reconstruction with dual plating.

macroscopic tumor, local adjuvants work primarily to eradicate the remaining microscopic tumor cells. Historically, liquid nitrogen was carefully poured directly into the bone cavity after curettage was completed.[62] The mechanism of cell death produced by liquid nitrogen cryotherapy involves a process of freezing and thawing, resulting in mechanical disruption of cellular membranes, ischemia, and induction of apoptosis.[63,64] When properly indicated, patients undergoing intralesional treatment with adjuvants have satisfactory outcomes. More recently, an argon-helium cryotherapy system has been used as an adjuvant treatment.[64] Complications associated with these adjuvant treatments have been reported to occur anywhere from 2% to 25% depending on the substance used.[64,65] Complications include fracture, damage to nearby structures, paresthesias, and infection. To enhance the integrity of the bone following local adjuvant treatment, substances such as autograft or allograft bone, polymethylmethacrylate, and other calcium-based synthetic materials can be used to fill the defect.[61]

Systemic adjuvants or neoadjuvants are also common depending on the specific pathology of the lesion, as such it is critical for patients to be evaluated by a multidisciplinary team to optimize outcomes. For example, treatment of osteosarcoma involves both neoadjuvant and adjuvant chemotherapy, so consultation with medical oncology is necessary for those patients. Some primary sarcomas are radiosensitive and radiation oncology should be consulted to be part of their multidisciplinary care team if this is the case. Patients with metastatic malignancies requiring prophylactic stabilization may benefit from undergoing postoperative radiotherapy and coordination of this care can be done while the patient is hospitalized.

EVALUATION OF OUTCOME AND/OR LONG-TERM RECOMMENDATIONS

There are numerous studies with small sample sizes from individual institutions reporting outcomes from various time points for all of the aforementioned surgical techniques. There remains no true standard or definitive indication for many of the specific techniques. Much of the decision to perform a certain type of reconstruction has to do with surgeon preference or institutional preference. Potter and colleagues[66] compared patients undergoing osteoarticular allograft, APC or endoprosthesis for a proximal humerus oncologic lesion at a median of 98 months. They reported that osteoarticular

allografts were most likely to require revision surgery, instability was more common in patients who had undergone an endoprosthesis, and APCs had the highest MSTS scores at 79% (compared with 71% for osteoarticular allograft and 69% for endoprosthesis). This group concluded that APCs should be offered to younger patients with primary sarcoma and endoprostheses would be a better option for older patients with metastases. Henderson and colleagues[39] performed a literature review and found that for 237 proximal humerus endoprosthetic cases, 33% resulted in failure. The complication rate of RSA for proximal humerus tumor is quite variable. Bonnevialle and colleagues[67] reported 38% unstable RSA prostheses at mean 42-month follow-up. At intermediate-term follow-up, one of nine patients had aseptic loosening of their RSA prosthesis in another study.[68] A 5-year outcome study for patients undergoing APC with hemiarthroplasty sought to determine if the early, 1-year outcomes persist at the 5-year mark. This series showed that the MSTS scores were worsening over time and forward elevation of the arm was decreased at 5 years compared with 1 year postoperatively, which they speculated is partially a result of superior humeral head migration.[69] Ten percent of the patients in that study were revised at the 5-year mark.

In an effort to more directly compare the outcomes the modern techniques of reconstruction for proximal humerus lesions, Houdek and colleagues[24] reviewed a cohort of 83 patients which included both hemiarthroplasty and RSA, endoprostheses and APCs. This cohort of patients over an 18-year period follows the trend toward RSA as the preferred technique that became prevalent at the institution. In terms of functional outcomes, RSA (both APC and endoprosthesis) had significantly better forward flexion and external rotation compared with hemiarthroplasty (APC and endoprosthesis). Patients with a hemiarthroplasty were more likely to subluxate compared with patients with an RSA. There were no differences in infection, reoperation, or revision procedures. Patient-reported outcome scores were also improved for patients with an RSA compared with patients with a hemiarthroplasty. Similarly, Zuo and colleagues[70] compared groups of patients undergoing APC hemiarthroplasty versus APC reverse total shoulder arthroplasty with a mean follow-up of 30 months. They reported better range of motion in the reverse arthroplasty group as well as better patient-reported outcomes in the form of ASES score compared with the hemiarthroplasty group.

Stress shielding is a term that describes the resorption of bone around the stem as the typical stresses on the bone are transferred to the implant.[71] Studies have reported as high as 92% of cohorts of cementless endoprostheses having evidence of stress shielding on x-ray.[71] Braig and colleagues[72] found that patients undergoing cemented modular endoprosthesis reconstruction of the proximal humerus had an incidence of stress shielding of 23%. Patients with stress shielding in their series had shorter implant stems and longer extramedullary components compared with those patients without stress shielding. Importantly, the clinical significance of stress shielding remains unknown, as the presence of stress shielding at mean follow-up of 5 ± 3 years did not predict failure of the implant.

SUMMARY/DISCUSSION/FUTURE DIRECTIONS

In summary, the proximal humerus is one of the most common location for both primary and metastatic oncologic lesions and there are numerous management strategies currently used in practice. The technology for the implants has improved in recent years as has the science behind adjuvant treatments that allow these patients to survive longer. As an example, a study of patients whose index surgery was before 1999 revealed abduction of no more than 45°,[73] which contrasts with more recent data reporting patients are able to reach a tall shelf and comb their hair without issue.[54] Currently, there are no standard procedures for specific proximal humerus tumors. Teunis and colleagues[59] discussed that there are many barriers to randomized controlled trials, most obviously that a power analysis revealed nearly 1000 patients would be the necessary sample size for an adequate trial which would likely require a large multi-center study. For now, smaller cohort studies continue to be published comparing the modern techniques and more specific groups of patients, which may help tease out what factors allow patients who have excellent outcomes and others to fail.

There are few studies that present data for customized patient-specific guides or implants for the indication of oncologic reconstruction at this time; however, this is likely a future direction in proximal humerus oncologic reconstruction. In general, outcomes for the procedures we currently use for proximal humerus tumors do not give consistently satisfactory outcomes and therefore there is work to be done to perfect these techniques and implants.

CLINICS CARE POINTS

- Intramedullary nail and open reduction and internal fixation with plate and cementation are valuable strategies for fixation of impending or complete pathologic fractures of the proximal humerus, particularly in the setting of metastatic disease.
- Although osteoarticular allografts and shoulder arthrodesis have fallen out of favor, vascularized fibula constructs can be instrumental for segmental bony defects (diaphyseal/metaphyseal).
- Hemiarthroplasty constructs for both endoprostheses and allograft prosthetic composite (APCs) have been recently reported to afford inferior outcomes for patients in terms of function and increased complications such as dislocation when compared with reverse shoulder arthroplasty (RSA) constructs though this is not necessarily standard and depends on surgeon preference among other factors.
- Both endoprosthetic and APC RSA constructs have shown encouraging results. APC constructs may have more utility in young patients and those with resections distal to the deltoid attachment.

DISCLOSURE

Dr. Barlow recieves consulting and royalty compensation from Stryker.

REFERENCES

1. Lee DH, Hills JM, Jordanov MI, et al. Common Tumors and Tumor-like Lesions of the Shoulder. J Am Acad Orthop Surg 2019;27(7):236–45.
2. Mascard E, Gomez-Brouchet A, Lambot K. Bone cysts: unicameral and aneurysmal bone cyst. Orthop Traumatol Surg Res 2015;101(1 Suppl): S119–27.
3. Wisanuyotin T, Sirichativapee W, Sumnanoont C, et al. Prognostic and risk factors in patients with metastatic bone disease of an upper extremity. J Bone Oncol 2018;13:71–5.
4. Voskuil RT, Mayerson JL, Scharschmidt TJ. Management of Metastatic Disease of the Upper Extremity. J Am Acad Orthop Surg 2021;29(3):e116–25.
5. Arpornsuksant P, Morris CD, Forsberg JA, et al. What Factors Are Associated With Local Metastatic Lesion Progression After Intramedullary Nail Stabilization? Clin Orthop Relat Res 2022;480(5):932–45.

6. Frassica FJ, Frassica DA. Evaluation and treatment of metastases to the humerus. Clin Orthop Relat Res 2003;(415 Suppl):S212–8.

7. Bickels J, Dadia S, Lidar Z. Surgical management of metastatic bone disease. J Bone Joint Surg Am 2009;91(6):1503–16.

8. Hu H, Liu W, Zeng Q, et al. The Personalized Shoulder Reconstruction Assisted by 3D Printing Technology After Resection of the Proximal Humerus Tumours. Cancer Manag Res 2019;11:10665–73.

9. Aparisi Gómez MP, Aparisi F, Battista G, et al. Functional and Surgical Anatomy of the Upper Limb: What the Radiologist Needs to Know. Radiol Clin North Am 2019;57(5):857–81.

10. Hakim DN, Pelly T, Kulendran M, et al. Benign tumours of the bone: A review. J bone Oncol 2015; 4(2):37–41.

11. Costelloe CM, Madewell JE. Radiography in the initial diagnosis of primary bone tumors. AJR Am J Roentgenol 2013;200(1):3–7.

12. Rougraff BT, Kneisl JS, Simon MA. Skeletal metastases of unknown origin. A prospective study of a diagnostic strategy. J Bone Joint Surg Am 1993; 75(9):1276–81.

13. Hennessy DW, Raskin KA, Schwab JH, et al. Endoprosthetic Reconstruction of the Upper Extremity in Oncologic Surgery. J Am Acad Orthop Surg 2020; 28(8):e319–27.

14. Bristow AR, Agrawal A, Evans AJ, et al. Can computerised tomography replace bone scintigraphy in detecting bone metastases from breast cancer? A prospective study. Breast 2008;17(1):98–103.

15. Malawer MM. Tumors of the shoulder girdle. Technique of resection and description of a surgical classification. Orthop Clin North Am 1991;22(1):7–35.

16. Wittig JC, Bickels J, Kellar-Graney KL, et al. Osteosarcoma of the proximal humerus: long-term results with limb-sparing surgery. Clin Orthop Relat Res 2002;397:156–76.

17. Alvi HM, Damron TA. Prophylactic stabilization for bone metastases, myeloma, or lymphoma: do we need to protect the entire bone? Clin Orthop Relat Res 2013;471(3):706–14.

18. Thai DM, Kitagawa Y, Choong PF. Outcome of surgical management of bony metastases to the humerus and shoulder girdle: a retrospective analysis of 93 patients. Int Semin Surg Oncol 2006;3:5.

19. MIRELS H. Metastatic Disease in Long Bones A Proposed Scoring System for Diagnosing Impending Pathologic Fractures. Clin Orthop Relat Res 1989; 249:256–64.

20. Evans AR, Bottros J, Grant W, et al. Mirels' rating for humerus lesions is both reproducible and valid. Clin Orthop Relat Res 2008;466(6):1279–84.

21. Miller BJ, Soni EE, Gibbs CP, et al. Intramedullary nails for long bone metastases: why do they fail? Orthopedics 2011;34(4).

22. Janssen SJ, Bramer JAM, Guitton TG, et al. Management of metastatic humeral fractures: Variations according to orthopedic subspecialty, tumor characteristics. Orthop Traumatol Surg Res 2018; 104(1):59–65.

23. Choi ES, Han I, Cho HS, et al. Intramedullary Nailing for Pathological Fractures of the Proximal Humerus. Clin Orthop Surg 2016;8(4):458–64.

24. Houdek MT, Bukowski BR, Athey AG, et al. Comparison of reconstructive techniques following oncologic intraarticular resection of proximal humerus. J Surg Oncol 2021;123(1):133–40.

25. Garg S, Sobol K, Munn M, et al. Effect of Radiation Field Size and Dose on Local Control or Re-fracture Events after Postoperative Radiation Following Intramedullary Nailing Procedures for Palliation of Bone Metastases. Int J Radiat Oncol Biol Phys 2018;102(3):e439–40.

26. Siegel HJ, Lopez-Ben R, Mann JP, et al. Pathological fractures of the proximal humerus treated with a proximal humeral locking plate and bone cement. J Bone Joint Surg Br 2010;92(5):707–12.

27. Wilson WT, Pickup AR, Findlay H, et al. Stabilisation of pathological humerus fractures using cement augmented plating: A case series. J Clin Orthop Trauma 2021;15:93–8.

28. SIM FH, DAUGHERTY TW, IVINS JC. The Adjunctive Use of Methylmethacrylate in Fixation of Pathological Fractures. JBJS 1974;56(1):40–8.

29. Weiss KR, Bhumbra R, Biau DJ, et al. Fixation of pathological humeral fractures by the cemented plate technique. J Bone Joint Surg Br 2011;93(8): 1093–7.

30. Hriscu M, Mojallal A, Breton P, et al. Limb salvage in proximal humerus malignant tumors: the place of free vascularized fibular graft. J Reconstr Microsurg 2006;22(6):415–21.

31. Fuchs B, O'Connor MI, Padgett DJ, et al. Arthrodesis of the shoulder after tumor resection. Clin Orthop Relat Res 2005;436:202–7.

32. Bilgin SS. Reconstruction of proximal humeral defects with shoulder arthrodesis using free vascularized fibular graft. J Bone Joint Surg Am 2012;94(13): e94.

33. Claxton MR, Shirley MB, Bakri K, et al. Utility of the Free Vascularized Fibula Flap to Reconstruct Oncologic Defects in the Upper Extremity. Anticancer Res 2020;40(5):2751–5.

34. Claxton MR, Houdek MT, Tibbo ME, et al. Utility of free vascularized fibular flaps to treat radiation-associated nonunions in the upper extremity. J Plast Reconstr Aesthet Surg 2020;73(4):633–7.

35. Campanacci DA, Totti F, Puccini S, et al. Intercalary reconstruction of femur after tumour resection: is a vascularized fibular autograft plus allograft a long-lasting solution? Bone Joint J 2018;100-b(3): 378–86.

36. DeGroot H, Donati D, Di Liddo M, et al. The use of cement in osteoarticular allografts for proximal humeral bone tumors. Clin Orthop Relat Res 2004; 427:190–7.

37. O'Connor MI, Sim FH, Chao EY. Limb salvage for neoplasms of the shoulder girdle. Intermediate reconstructive and functional results. J Bone Joint Surg Am 1996;78(12):1872–88.

38. Rödl RW, Gosheger G, Gebert C, et al. Reconstruction of the proximal humerus after wide resection of tumours. J Bone Joint Surg Br 2002;84(7):1004–8.

39. Henderson ER, Groundland JS, Pala E, et al. Failure mode classification for tumor endoprostheses: retrospective review of five institutions and a literature review. J Bone Joint Surg Am 2011;93(5):418–29.

40. Damron TA, Rock MG, O'Connor MI, et al. Functional Laboratory Assessment After Oncologic Shoulder Joint Resections. Clin Orthop Relat Res 1998;348:124–34.

41. Fuhrmann RA, Roth A, Venbrocks RA. Salvage of the upper extremity in cases of tumorous destruction of the proximal humerus. J Cancer Res Clin Oncol 2000;126(6):337–44.

42. Cundy WJ, McArthur MS, Dickinson IC, et al. Constrained or unconstrained shoulder replacement for musculoskeletal tumor resections? J Shoulder Elbow Surg 2020;29(10):2104–10.

43. Maclean S, Malik SS, Evans S, et al. Reverse shoulder endoprosthesis for pathologic lesions of the proximal humerus: a minimum 3-year follow-up. J Shoulder Elbow Surg 2017;26(11):1990–4.

44. Chalmers PN, Keener JD. Expanding roles for reverse shoulder arthroplasty. Curr Rev Musculoskelet Med 2016;9(1):40–8.

45. Ackland DC, Patel M, Knox D. Prosthesis design and placement in reverse total shoulder arthroplasty. J Orthop Surg Res 2015;10:101.

46. Grosel TW, Plummer DR, Mayerson JL, et al. Oncologic reconstruction of the proximal humerus with a reverse total shoulder arthroplasty megaprosthesis. J Surg Oncol 2018;118(6):867–72.

47. Flury MP, Frey P, Goldhahn J, et al. Reverse shoulder arthroplasty as a salvage procedure for failed conventional shoulder replacement due to cuff failure–midterm results. Int Orthop 2011;35(1):53–60.

48. Elhassan BT, Wagner ER, Werthel JD, et al. Outcome of reverse shoulder arthroplasty with pedicled pectoralis transfer in patients with deltoid paralysis. J Shoulder Elbow Surg 2018;27(1):96–103.

49. Ayvaz M, Cetik RM, Bakircioglu S, et al. Proximal Humerus Tumors: Higher-than-Expected Risk of Revision With Constrained Reverse Shoulder Arthroplasty. Clin Orthop Relat Res 2020;478(11):2585–95.

50. Takahashi T, Sato T, Manabe J, et al. Reverse shoulder arthroplasty and synthetic mesh for reconstruction of the shoulder joint after malignant bone tumor resection: A case report. Med Case Rep Study Protoc 2021;2(2):e0051.

51. Marulanda GA, Henderson E, Cheong D, et al. Proximal and total humerus reconstruction with the use of an aortograft mesh. Clin Orthop Relat Res 2010;468(11):2896–903.

52. Raiss P, Kinkel S, Sauter U, et al. Replacement of the proximal humerus with MUTARS tumor endoprostheses. Eur J Surg Oncol 2010;36(4):371–7.

53. van de Sande MA, Dijkstra PD, Taminiau AH. Proximal humerus reconstruction after tumour resection: biological versus endoprosthetic reconstruction. Int Orthop 2011;35(9):1375–80.

54. Tang X, Guo W, Yang R, et al. Synthetic mesh improves shoulder function after intraarticular resection and prosthetic replacement of proximal humerus. Clin Orthop Relat Res 2015;473(4):1464–71.

55. Degeorge B, Chammas M, Coulet B, et al. Allograft-Composite Reverse Shoulder Arthroplasty for Malignant Tumor of the Proximal Humerus. Tech Hand Up Extrem Surg 2020;25(2):94–101.

56. Sanchez-Sotelo J, Wagner ER, Houdek MT. Allograft-Prosthetic Composite Reconstruction for Massive Proximal Humeral Bone Loss in Reverse Shoulder Arthroplasty. JBJS Essent Surg Tech 2018;8(1):e3–.

57. Sanchez-Sotelo J, Wagner ER, Sim FH, et al. Allograft-Prosthetic Composite Reconstruction for Massive Proximal Humeral Bone Loss in Reverse Shoulder Arthroplasty. J Bone Joint Surg Am 2017;99(24):2069–76.

58. King JJ, Nystrom LM, Reimer NB, et al. Allograft-prosthetic composite reverse total shoulder arthroplasty for reconstruction of proximal humerus tumor resections. J Shoulder Elbow Surg 2016; 25(1):45–54.

59. Teunis T, Nota SP, Hornicek FJ, et al. Outcome after reconstruction of the proximal humerus for tumor resection: a systematic review. Clin Orthop Relat Res 2014;472(7):2245–53.

60. Zou Y, Yang Y, Han Q, et al. Novel exploration of customized 3D printed shoulder prosthesis in revision of total shoulder arthroplasty: A case report. Medicine 2018;97(47):e13282.

61. Veth R, Schreuder B, van Beem H, et al. Cryosurgery in aggressive, benign, and low-grade malignant bone tumours. Lancet Oncol 2005;6(1):25–34.

62. Marcove RC, Miller TR. Treatment of primary and metastatic bone tumors by cryosurgery. Jama 1969;207(10):1890–4.

63. Gage AA, Baust JG. Cryosurgery - a review of recent advances and current issues. Cryo Lett 2002;23(2):69–78.

64. Yang Y, Han L, He Z, et al. Advances in limb salvage treatment of osteosarcoma. J Bone Oncol 2018;10: 36–40.

65. Chen C, Garlich J, Vincent K, et al. Postoperative complications with cryotherapy in bone tumors. J Bone Oncol 2017;7:13–7.

66. Potter BK, Adams SC, Pitcher JD Jr. Malinin TI, Temple HT. Proximal humerus reconstructions for tumors. Clin Orthop Relat Res 2009;467(4): 1035–41.

67. Bonnevialle N, Mansat P, Lebon J, et al. Reverse shoulder arthroplasty for malignant tumors of proximal humerus. J Shoulder Elbow Surg 2015;24(1): 36–44.

68. De Wilde L, Boileau P, Van der Bracht H. Does Reverse Shoulder Arthroplasty for Tumors of the Proximal Humerus Reduce Impairment? Clin Orthop Relat Res 2011;469(9):2489–95.

69. El Beaino M, Liu J, Lewis VO, et al. Do Early Results of Proximal Humeral Allograft-Prosthetic Composite Reconstructions Persist at 5-year Followup? Clin Orthop Relat Res 2019;477(4):758–65.

70. Zuo D, Mu H, Yang Q, et al. Do reverse total shoulder replacements have better clinical and functional outcomes than hemiarthroplasty for patients undergoing proximal humeral tumor resection using devitalized autograft composite reconstruction: a case-control study. J Orthop Surg Res 2021;16(1):453.

71. Klingebiel S, Schneider KN, Gosheger G, et al. Periprosthetic Stress Shielding of the Humerus after Reconstruction with Modular Shoulder Megaprostheses in Patients with Sarcoma. J Clin Med 2021;10(15).

72. Braig ZV, Tagliero AJ, Rose PS, et al. Humeral stress shielding following cemented endoprosthetic reconstruction: An under-reported complication? J Surg Oncol 2021;123(2):505–9.

73. Kumar D, Grimer RJ, Abudu A, et al. Endoprosthetic replacement of the proximal humerus. Long-term results. J Bone Joint Surg Br 2003; 85(5):717–22.

Management of Scapular Tumors

Matthew T. Houdek, MD[a,*], Benjamin K. Wilke, MD[b], Jonathan D. Barlow, MD[a]

KEYWORDS

- Scapulectomy • Tikhoff-Linberg • Shoulder girdle

KEY POINTS

- Limb salvage surgery
- Upper extremity sarcoma
- Proximal humerus sarcoma

INTRODUCTION

The scapula forms the posterior shoulder girdle and is essential for function, acting as the origin or insertion for 17 different muscles.[1,2] It is responsible for 6 types of motion, allowing for a functional upper extremity including elevation, depression, upward and downward rotation, protraction, and retraction.[1,2] Because of the critical function of the scapula, limb salvage procedures are preferred as an alternative to forequarter amputation.

Scapular resections have advanced since the first reported partial scapulectomy performed in 1819 by Liston.[3] Scapular resections were then limited to small series and case reports, and in 1909 De Nancrede concluded that anything less than a forequarter amputation for a shoulder girdle tumor was inadequate.[4] Interscapulothoracic resection offered a limb salvage approach to patients with scapular tumors, and was first described by Bauman in Russian and then Tikhoff and Linberg in English;[5,6] however, these resections were felt to potentially put the patient at high risk of recurrence secondary to the proximity of the brachial plexus and axillary vessels. Because of this, forequarter amputations were performed for many patients with large tumors involving the scapula until the 1970s. With advances in medical imaging, neoadjuvant treatments, and surgical techniques, limb salvage surgery has become the preferred surgical technique, allowing for an oncologic margin while preserving hand function.[7–9]

PATIENT EVALUATION

Like other types of sarcomas, patients with a primary bone sarcoma of the scapula often present with a mass and pain, while patients with a soft-tissue sarcoma often present with a painless, enlarging mass. Because the scapula is surrounded by multiple muscles, masses can get quite large before presentation. In the scapula, the most common bony sarcomas are chondrosarcomas in adults and Ewing sarcoma in children and adolescents.[10]

A limb salvage surgery is contraindicated if the brachial plexus is involved and resection of the portions of the brachial plexus would lead to a nonfunctional hand that is not amenable to nerve or muscle transfer. Clinically, involvement of the brachial plexus can be suspected if there is intractable pain and motor deficits. In the initial work up of patients involves plain film radiographs and cross-sectional imaging consisting of an MRI with contrast and computed tomography (CT) scan of the chest. It is important to obtain an MRI that includes the entire chest, axilla, glenohumeral joint, and neck to evaluate the brachial plexus for tumor extension. In addition, a CT-angiogram and

[a] Department of Orthopedic Surgery, Mayo Clinic, Rochester, MN, USA; [b] Department of Orthopedic Surgery, Mayo Clinic, Jacksonville, FL, USA
* Corresponding author. 200 First Street Southwest, Rochester, MN 55905.
E-mail address: houdek.matthew@mayo.edu

Orthop Clin N Am 54 (2023) 101–108
https://doi.org/10.1016/j.ocl.2022.08.009

venogram are important to evaluate the axillary and subclavian vein, as obliteration of the vein can indicate involvement of the axillary sheath and subsequent involvement of the brachial plexus.

BIOPSY

If a sarcoma is suspected, a carefully planned needle biopsy is essential. It is important that the biopsy is performed under the guidance of the team that will ultimately be treating the patient, as an inappropriately placed biopsy could lead to an amputation.[11] Since scapular sarcomas often present with a large soft-tissue mass; a needle biopsy is often able to obtain lesional tissue. The biopsy should be performed posteriorly in line with the planned incision. Anterior biopsies should be avoided, if possible, to avoid contamination of the neurovascular structures. If the tumor is located in the scapular neck or glenoid, the biopsy should be placed through the posterior deltoid and teres minor.

Staging of Patients

Once a sarcoma is diagnosed patients should be staged based on tumor histology. For soft-tissue sarcomas, the patient requires a CT scan of the chest to evaluate for metastatic disease. For bone sarcomas, patients require a CT scan of the chest and either a whole-body bone scan or PET-CT scan for osteosarcomas or Ewing sarcomas. A bone scan or PET-CT is not required for chondrosarcoma unless a de-differentiated chondrosarcoma is diagnosed on the preoperative biopsy.[12,13] In addition a bone-marrow biopsy is not required in patients with a Ewing sarcoma if there are no signs metastatic disease on other staging studies.[14,15]

Once the patient has been staged, referral to medical oncology and radiation oncology is essential for the treatment of patients in a multidisciplinary fashion. Treatment is individualized and based on tumor histology. For patients with a Ewing sarcoma, interval compressed chemotherapy consisting of vincristine-doxorubicin-cyclophosphamide and ifosfamide-etoposide (VDC/IE) combined with surgical resection has improved survival.[16,17] For patients with osteosarcoma, the standard treatment involves neoadjuvant chemotherapy, surgical resection, and adjuvant chemotherapy with the chemotherapy backbone including methotrexate, doxorubicin, and cisplatin (MAP).[18] For patients with chondrosarcoma, surgery is the only option for management, as these tumors are resistant to chemotherapy and

radiotherapy.[18] Because patients with soft-tissue sarcoma involving the scapula often present with deep, large, high-grade tumors, a combination of radiotherapy and surgical resection has become the standard treatment.[19] Chemotherapy is typically not combined for treatment of patients with soft-tissue sarcomas, as the use of chemotherapy has not been shown to improve survival when combined with radiotherapy and surgery.[20]

Surgical Resection

With the adoption of limb salvage surgery for patients with malignancies involving the shoulder girdle, different classification systems were developed to quantify the magnitude of the resection and the preservation of critical soft tissue structures. Currently the Malawer classification system and Musculoskeletal Tumor Society (MSTS) Classification of Skeletal Resections (Fig. 1) are the most utilized classification systems.[5,21] Both systems stratify by location of the resection and the status of the deltoid and the rotator cuff, as preservation of the glenohumeral joint has been found to be most impactful on functional outcomes.[5,21]

Patients with sarcomas of the scapula are managed with the patient in a rolling lateral position, to allow access to the posterior and anterior shoulder girdle. This should include the

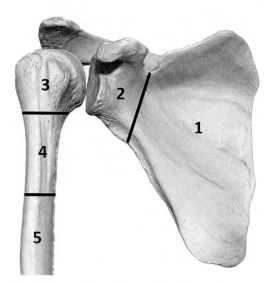

Fig. 1. Anatomic breakdown of shoulder gridle resections based on the MSTS system. The Tikhoff-Linberg classification is based on similar anatomic structures and would include Type 1: (3, 4, 5); Type 2: (1); Type 3: (1, 2); Type IV: (1, 2, 3); Type V: (2, 3, 4, 5); Type IV: (1, 2, 3, 4, 5). Both systems also include the status of the deltoid and rotator cuff, as either being intact (A) or deficient (B).

ipsilateral arm and neck, and the prep should extend past midline on the chest and back.

TOTAL SCAPULAR RESECTIONS

For patients who require resection of the entire scapula, (Fig. 2) or if the resection includes the proximal humerus, a utilitarian incision is utilized. This incision starts as an extended deltopectoral approach and extends proximally over the clavicle, curving posterior along the lateral border of the latissimus and then turning toward the inferior portion of the scapula and midline. The anterior portion of the incision should be explored first to evaluate if the brachial plexus and axillary vessels can be freed of the tumor. The pectoralis major is released from the humerus and retracted medial. The conjoint tendon and pectoralis minor are released from the coracoid, keeping a cuff of tendon on the coracoid. This allows exposure of the brachial plexus and vessels. The short head of the biceps is released distal to the subscapularis tendon at the level of the musculotendinous junction of the short-head of the biceps. It is important to carefully evaluate the preoperative MRI for tumor extension down the biceps tendon. This allows the biceps to be reflected medial, pulling the musculocutaneous nerve, allowing it to be protected. The shoulder can then be externally rotated, and the latissimus and teres major are reflected off the proximal humerus to expose the radial nerve. The anterior circumflex vessels are ligated, allowing the axillary artery and vein to fall medial. Often the axillary nerve can be salvaged and can be freed off the inferior joint capsule anteriorly, and then the dissection is completed during the posterior exposure.

Based on the tumor extent, the deltoid can be released off the clavicle, acromion and scapular spine. In the process of doing this posteriorly, the axillary nerve and posterior circumflex vessels can be visualized. If the deltoid can be preserved, the nerve and vessels are kept in continuity with the muscle belly by freeing them from the underlying capsule, in addition by ligating the branches headed to the teres minor. The incision is then turned posterior and along the lateral boarder of the latissimus, curving toward the inferior angle of the scapula. Large skin flaps are created, and the trapezius and triceps are released from the scapula. It is important to evaluate the extent of the tumor in relation to the chest wall, as a portion of the serratus anterior muscle can often be preserved; however, if there is concern for tumor involvement, the serratus anterior should be included in the resection. The shoulder can then be internally rotated and the patient's hand placed behind the iliac crest in a figure-4 fashion. This pushes the tip of the scapula away from the chest wall, allowing for medial periscapular muscles to be reflected off the scapula. This is carried from an inferior to superior fashion, allowing the scapula to be everted away from the chest wall. Once this is completed, the clavicle can be osteotomized or the acromioclavicular joint is disarticulated,

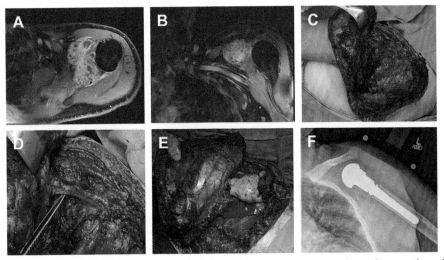

Fig. 2. Axial (A) and coronal (B) MRI with contrast showing a chondrosarcoma involving the scapula and glenoid. The patient underwent an extra-articular resection of the proximal humerus and scapula through a utilitarian incision with the posterior limb of the incision (C) shown following scapular resection with preservation of axillary nerve (D). The proximal humerus was reconstructed using an endoprosthesis wrapped in mesh (E), which was suspended from the clavicle (F).

allowing for mobilization of the specimen. If there is a large anterior soft tissue mass, the scapula can be lifted off the chest wall posteriorly, exposing the axillary vessels from the back and allowing for easy ligation of the suprascapular vessels and a neurectomy of the suprascapular nerve. Once the soft tissues of the scapula are fully released, the proximal humerus can be cut distal based on the extent of the tumor in the setting of an extra-articular resection, or the rotator cuff can be sectioned at the insertion of the humeral head circumferentially in the setting of an intra-articular resection. If there is difficulty removing the specimen following the humeral cut, it is often secondary to the preservation of the coracoclavicular ligaments based on the level of the clavicular osteotomy.

The residual deltoid and trapezius are repaired to any residual clavicle and can be tenodesed if there is no residual bone. It is important to use transosseous sutures if there is remaining clavicle. Based on the type of bony reconstruction, the residual soft tissues can be used to assist with closure, but also to restore function. The latissimus can be used to assist with external rotation by mobilizing it to a lateral, anterosuperior location on the residual humerus or implant.[22] Similarly, the lower trapezius can be mobilized to the lateral, posterosuperior residual humerus, or implant to assist with external rotation.[23] The wound should be closed in multiple layers over large suction drains. The patient should be kept in an abduction shoulder immobilizer for soft-tissue healing. Patients are allowed active, active-assisted, and passive range of motion of the elbow, hand, and wrist immediately following surgery; however, shoulder motion should avoided until 6 weeks postoperatively. At that time, patients are allowed to begin stretching and deltoid retraining exercises.

PARTIAL SCAPULECTOMY

Partial scapular resections are typically performed from a posterior approach (Fig. 3), unless a portion of the glenoid needs to be resected along with a proximal humeral resection. For posterior approaches to the scapula, the patient is positioned in a rolling lateral position with the arm and neck included in the sterile field. The approach to the scapula is performed utilizing the posterior portion of the utilitarian approach used for total scapular resections. The incision can either be a "J" incision starting from approximately a hand's breath from the

lateral tip of the acromion and extending distally along the border of the latissimus before curving toward the tip of the scapula, or a diagonal incision extending from the tip of the scapula to the glenohumeral joint. The authors' preferred incision is a "J" incision, as it can be extended anteriorly in case the anterior neurovascular structures need to be explored.

Large skin flaps are elevated during exposure, and often the trapezius can be preserved. The deltoid is reflected off the scapular spine, exposing the underlying scapula. The latissimus is pulled inferior, exposing the serratus insertion. The shoulder can be internally rotated, and the patient's hand placed behind the iliac crest in a Fig. 4 fashion. This pushes the tip of the scapula away from the chest wall, allowing for the medial periscapular muscles to be reflected off the scapula. This is carried from an inferior to superior fashion, allowing the scapula to be everted off the chest wall. The lateral border of the scapula is then exposed by reflecting the teres and triceps, exposing the underlying neurovascular bundles. Branches entering the tumor are ligated, allowing the axillary nerve and posterior circumflex vessels to fall lateral. Once the scapula is completely exposed, the scapular osteotomy can be performed based on the tumor extent. The infraspinatus and the supraspinatus tendons can be released directly off the humerus, keeping a cuff of muscle on the tumor specimen. The supraspinatus will need to be released from a posterior to anterior fashion. The serratus is then released from the under surface of the scapula, allowing the surgeon to be able to pass his or her hand under the entire scapula, allowing for a tactile sense of where to create the osteotomy. The authors' preference is to utilize a harmonic scalpel to cut from a posterior to anterior fashion. The soft tissues of the subscapularis are then divided. This allows for the specimen to be rotated off the chest wall, exposing any neurovascular structures entering the specimen that can then be carefully ligated allowing for the specimen to be delivered from the field.

A soft-tissue only repair is frequently performed by suturing the residual deltoid and trapezius to any residual scapula, or these muscles may be tenodesed if there is no residual scapula. Any residual rotator cuff should also be sutured together, and the teres can be tenodesed to the latissimus to assist with rotation. The wound is closed in multiple layers over large suction drains, and the patient is kept in a shoulder immobilizer for soft-tissue healing. Patients

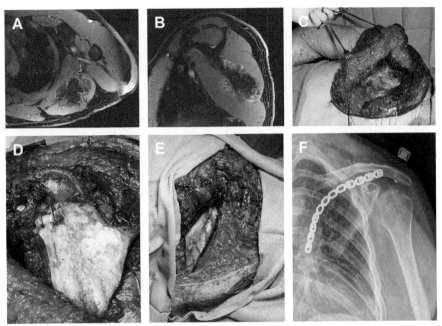

Fig. 3. Axial (*A*) and sagittal (*B*) MRI with contrast showing a secondary chondrosarcoma involving the inferior aspect of the scapula. The patient underwent a partial scapulectomy from a posterior approach (*C*). The scapula was reconstructed with an allograft (*D*) and soft-tissue reconstruction was performed with a lower trapezial (*E*) transfer with healing of allograft (*F*) at most recent follow-up.

are allowed to be active, active assisted, andpassive range of motion of the elbow, hand, and wrist immediately following surgery; however, shoulder motion is avoided until 4 weeks postoperatively. At that time patients are allowed to begin stretching and deltoid retraining exercises.

CURETTAGE

Extended intralesional curettage should only be used in the setting of a biopsy-confirmed benign aggressive tumors or in the setting of symptomatic metastatic disease on a case-by-case basis. In this setting, a combined approach of curettage and adjuvants including thermal, mechanical, and chemical, provides local tumor control. The authors' preferred technique is to use a high-speed burr, hydrogen peroxide, and an argon beam electrocoagulator.

Reconstruction

The necessity of reconstruction following scapulectomy is a debated topic. For patients with partial scapulectomy, only a soft-tissue closure is necessary, and the patient should expect near normal function. If the glenoid is resected, the functional outcomes are inferior compared to if the glenoid and deltoid are preserved.[24–26] If the glenoid is resected, often reconstruction can be performed with an augmented reverse

total shoulder base plate, combined proximal humerus allograft, and free vascularized fibula for arthrodesis, or suspension of the proximal humerus based on the extent of bony and soft-tissue resection.[27] Following partial scapular resection, complications are associated with the extent of soft tissue resection and involve mainly wound complications and subluxation of an implant if is one is utilized.[24–27]

For patients who have had a total scapular resection, in addition to the proximal humerus, series have shown the use of a scapular prosthesis, or an allograft scapula combined with a scapular thoracic arthrodesis, can return some shoulder function in selected patients.[28–30] In limited series, the use of a scapular endoprosthesis could provide improvements in shoulder range of motion and functional outcomes: however, similar to partial scapular resection, functional outcomes are based on the amount of soft tissue preserved following tumor resection. If there is not sufficient soft tissue, a functional spacer of the proximal humerus suspended from the chest wall or residual clavicle can allow for a stable platform for elbow, wrist, and hand motion.[31] Complications remain high following reconstruction for total scapular resection and are most commonly secondary to wound complications and related to the use of neoadjuvant radiotherapy.[29,31] In addition to wound

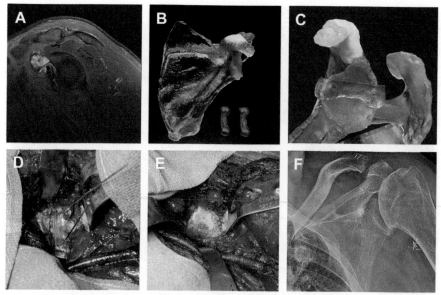

Fig. 4. Sagittal T2 (*A*) MRI showing a low-grade chondrosarcoma involving the coracoid. In order to reduce the size of resection, a 3-dimensional model and patient-specific guides were fabricated (*B*) to allow for an osteotomy of the coracoid from the glenoid (*C*). The guide was placed intraoperatively (*D*), and the cut (*E*) allowed for a negative margin excision and preservation of most of the glenoid (*F*).

complications, prosthetic complications associated with a humeral suspension include subluxation of the implant and stress shielding.[32]

New Developments

Similar to other areas in orthopedics, the use of custom implants for reconstruction of complex oncologic resections has become a new option for surgeons following scapular resection.[33–35] Although there is promise that these patient-specific implants could allow for functional recovery following scapulectomy, the results of these studies are limited to small series and case reports. In addition to custom implants, 3-dimensional printed cutting guides and anatomic models are allowing for smaller resections (see Fig. 4), and a partial scapular resection where previously larger resections were necessary to provide an appropriate oncologic margin.[36]

Patient Follow-Up

Following oncologic resection, patients should follow-up routinely with the orthopedic and medical oncology teams based on the tumor histology. Follow-up involves physical examination and routine imaging. Radiographic imaging includes plain radiographs of the shoulder and pulmonary imaging consisting of a CT scan of the lungs, or a chest radiograph. The routine use of cross-sectional imaging of the operative site is debated, as a local recurrence can often

be detected by clinical examination alone.[37,38] At our institution for high-grade tumors, patients are followed every 3 to 4 months for the first 2 years postoperatively, every 6 months for years 2 to 5, and then annually for years 5 to 10. For low-grade tumors, follow-up is every 4 months for the first 2 years, every 6 months for year 3, and then annually for years 4 to 5. Following the completion of follow-up with the orthopedic oncology team for low- or high-grade tumors, it is recommended the patient follow-up with his or her primary care provider for periodic chest radiographs, as long-term metastatic disease has been reported.

Following oncologic resection, patients with scapular sarcomas have been thought to have improved oncologic outcomes compared with bone sarcomas located in other areas. In patients with scapular chondrosarcoma, previous series have demonstrated a low rate of recurrence;[26,39] however, these were limited because of their lack of patients with high-grade tumors. In patients with a greater portion of high-grade tumors involving the scapula, 10-year survival is between 50% to 80%, and is strongly associated with the grade of the tumor.[28,40,41] An important factor when treating patients with a scapular chondrosarcoma is to avoid any intralesional procedure. All scapular chondrosarcomas should be treated with wide local excision. Prior series have shown that patients who undergo an intralesional procedure are at increased risk of local recurrence, and that local tumor recurrence is associated with metastatic disease.[28]

SUMMARY

Scapular resections are large oncologic undertakings. Patient outcomes are strongly tied to the extent of resection, with the goal of surgery to provide a stable platform for elbow, hand, and wrist motion. Even though intralesional procedures have the potential to allow for a smaller resection, they should be avoided secondary to the risk of local recurrence and subsequent metastatic disease. Although there are options for scapular reconstruction, the use of endoprosthetic or allograft reconstruction of the scapula is limited to small case series with limited follow-up; as such, recommendations for reconstruction in all patients cannot be given.

CLINICS CARE POINTS

- Careful preoperative evaluation of the brachial plexus and axillary vessels is essential to determine if a limb salvage procedure can be performed. If two of the main nerves to the hand (median, radial, or ulnar) are involved and need to be resected, the patient's hand would be nonfunctional, and as such, a forequarter should be performed.

- In patients undergoing total scapular resection, the anterior limb of the incision should be performed first to evaluate the involvement of the brachial plexus and axillary vessels.

- Following oncologic resection, reconstructive options are limited in the setting of a total scapular resection. As such, the goals for reconstruction remain providing a stable platform for elbow, wrist, and hand use.

DISCLOSURE

The authors have no disclosures.

REFERENCES

1. Miniato MA, Mudreac A, Borger J. Anatomy, Thorax, Scapula. In: StatPearls. FL: Treasure Island; 2022.
2. Cowan PT, Mudreac A, Varacallo M. Anatomy, Back, Scapula. In: StatPearls. FL: Treasure ,Island; 2022.
3. Liston R. Ossified aneurysmal tumor of the subscapular artery. Eduil Med J 1820;16:66–70.
4. De Nancrede CBI. End results after total excision of the scapula for sarcoma: with statistical tables. Ann Surg 1909;50(1):1–22.
5. Malawer MM. Tumors of the shoulder girdle. Technique of resection and description of a surgical classification. Orthop Clin North Am 1991;22(1):7–35.
6. Linberg BE. Interscapulo-thoracic resection for malignant tumors of the shoulder joint region. Clin Orthop Relat Res 1928;1999(358):3–7.
7. Marcove RC, Lewis MM, Huvos AG. En bloc upper humeral interscapulo-thoracic resection. The Tikhoff-Linberg procedure. Clin Orthop Relat Res 1977;124:219–28.
8. Bickels J, Wittig JC, Kollender Y, et al. Limb-sparing resections of the shoulder girdle. J Am Coll Surg 2002;194(4):422–35.
9. O'Connor MI, Sim FH, Chao EY. Limb salvage for neoplasms of the shoulder girdle. Intermediate reconstructive and functional results. J Bone Joint Surg Am 1996;78(12):1872–88.
10. Kaiser CL, Yeung CM, Raskin K, et al. Tumors of the scapula: a retrospective analysis identifying predictors of malignancy. Surg Oncol 2020;32:18–22.
11. Mankin HJ, Mankin CJ, Simon MA. The hazards of the biopsy, revisited. Members of the Musculoskeletal Tumor Society. J Bone Joint Surg Am 1996; 78(5):656–63.
12. Johnson JD, Rainer WG, Rose PS, et al. Utility of bone scintigraphy and PET-CT in the surgical staging of skeletal chondrosarcoma. Anticancer Res 2020;40(10):5735–8.
13. Gulia A, Kurisunkal V, Puri A, et al. Is skeletal imaging essential in the staging workup for conventional chondrosarcoma? Clin Orthop Relat Res 2020; 478(11):2480–4.
14. Cesari M, Righi A, Colangeli M, et al. Bone marrow biopsy in the initial staging of Ewing sarcoma: experience from a single institution. Pediatr Blood Cancer 2019;66(6):e27653.
15. Kasalak O, Glaudemans A, Overbosch J, et al. Can FDG-PET/CT replace blind bone marrow biopsy of the posterior iliac crest in Ewing sarcoma? Skeletal Radiol 2018;47(3):363–7.
16. Leavey PJ, Laack NN, Krailo MD, et al. Phase III trial adding vincristine-topotecan-cyclophosphamide to the initial treatment of patients with nonmetastatic Ewing sarcoma: a Children's Oncology Group report. J Clin Oncol 2021;39(36):4029–38.
17. Womer RB, West DC, Krailo MD, et al. Randomized controlled trial of interval-compressed chemotherapy for the treatment of localized Ewing sarcoma: a report from the Children's Oncology Group. J Clin Oncol 2012;30(33):4148–54.
18. Strauss SJ, Frezza AM, Abecassis N, et al. Bone sarcomas: ESMO-EURACAN-GENTURIS-ERN

PaedCan Clinical Practice Guideline for diagnosis, treatment and follow-up. Ann Oncol 2021;32(12): 1520–36.

19. Gronchi A, Miah AB, Dei Tos AP, et al. Soft tissue and visceral sarcomas: ESMO-EURACAN-GENTURIS Clinical Practice Guidelines for diagnosis, treatment and follow-up. Ann Oncol 2021; 32(11):1348–65.

20. Pervaiz N, Colterjohn N, Farrokhyar F, et al. A systematic meta-analysis of randomized controlled trials of adjuvant chemotherapy for localized resectable soft-tissue sarcoma. Cancer 2008;113(3):573–81.

21. Enneking W, Dunham W, Gebhardt M, et al. A system for the classification of skeletal resections. Chir Organi Mov 1990;75(1 Suppl):217–40.

22. Elhassan BT, Wagner ER, Kany J. Latissimus dorsi transfer for irreparable subscapularis tear. J Shoulder Elbow Surg 2020;29(10):2128–34.

23. Elhassan BT, Sanchez-Sotelo J, Wagner ER. Outcome of arthroscopically assisted lower trapezius transfer to reconstruct massive irreparable posterior-superior rotator cuff tears. J Shoulder Elbow Surg 2020;29(10):2135–42.

24. Schwab JH, Athanasian EA, Morris CD, et al. Function correlates with deltoid preservation in patients having scapular replacement. Clin Orthop Relat Res 2006;452:225–30.

25. Damron TA, Rock MG, O'Connor MI, et al. Functional laboratory assessment after oncologic shoulder joint resections. Clin Orthop Relat Res 1998; 348:124–34.

26. Griffin AM, Shaheen M, Bell RS, et al. Oncologic and functional outcome of scapular chondrosarcoma. Ann Surg Oncol 2008;15(8):2250–6.

27. Houdek MT, Bukowski BR, Athey AG, et al. Comparison of reconstructive techniques following oncologic intraarticular resection of proximal humerus. J Surg Oncol 2021;123(1):133–40.

28. Wellings EP, Mallett KE, Parkes CW, et al. Impact of tumour stage on the surgical outcomes of scapular chondrosarcoma. Int Orthop 2022;46(5):1175–80.

29. Pritsch T, Bickels J, Wu CC, et al. Is scapular endoprosthesis functionally superior to humeral suspension? Clin Orthop Relat Res 2007;456:188–95.

30. Schoch B, Shives T, Elhassan B. Subtotal scapulectomy with scapulothoracic fusion and local tendon transfer for management of chondrosarcoma. J Am Acad Orthop Surg 2016;24(6):405–9.

31. Scorianz M, Houdek MT, Sherman CE, et al. Survival, tumor recurrence, and function following shoulder girdle limb salvage at 24 to 35 years of follow-up. Orthopedics 2019;42(6):e514–20.

32. Braig ZV, Tagliero AJ, Rose PS, et al. Humeral stress shielding following cemented endoprosthetic reconstruction: an under-reported complication? J Surg Oncol 2021;123(2):505–9.

33. Grossi S, D'Arienzo A, Sacchetti F, et al. One-step reconstruction with custom-made 3d-printed scapular prosthesis after partial or total scapulectomy. Surg Technol Int 2020;36:341–6.

34. Savvidou OD, Zampeli F, Georgopoulos G, et al. Total scapulectomy and shoulder reconstruction using a scapular prosthesis and constrained reverse shoulder arthroplasty. Orthopedics 2018;41(6):e888–93.

35. Beltrami G, Ristori G, Scocciianti G, et al. Latissimus dorsi rotational flap combined with a custom-made scapular prosthesis after oncological surgical resection: a report of two patients. BMC Cancer 2018; 18(1):1003.

36. Matsumoto JS, Morris JM, Rose PS. 3-dimensional printed anatomic models as planning aids in complex oncology surgery. JAMA Oncol 2016;2(9): 1121–2.

37. England P, Hong Z, Rhea L, et al. Does advanced imaging have a role in detecting local recurrence of soft-tissue sarcoma? Clin Orthop Relat Res 2020;478(12):2812–20.

38. Cipriano C, Griffin AM, Ferguson PC, et al. Developing an evidence-based follow-up schedule for bone sarcomas based on local recurrence and metastatic progression. Clin Orthop Relat Res 2017; 475(3):830–8.

39. Pant R, Yasko AW, Lewis VO, et al. Chondrosarcoma of the scapula: long-term oncologic outcome. Cancer 2005;104(1):149–58.

40. Nota SP, Russchen MJ, Raskin KA, et al. Functional and oncological outcome after surgical resection of the scapula and clavicle for primary chondrosarcoma. Musculoskelet Surg 2017;101(1):67–73.

41. Schneiderbauer MM, Blanchard C, Gullerud R, et al. Scapular chondrosarcomas have high rates of local recurrence and metastasis. Clin Orthop Relat Res 2004;426:232–8.

Foot and Ankle

Management of Periprosthetic Bone Cysts After Total Ankle Arthroplasty

Edward S. Hur, MD, Nabil Mehta, MD, Simon Lee, MD,
Daniel D. Bohl, MD, MPH*

KEYWORDS

- Total ankle arthroplasty • Bone cysts • Osteolysis • Revision arthroplasty

---

KEY POINTS

- Periprosthetic bone cysts are common after total ankle arthroplasty and can often be asymptomatic.
- The exact cause of bone cyst formation is likely multifactorial with contributing factors including polyethylene wear, implant micromotion, and implant design.
- Nonoperative management includes observation with annual clinical and radiographic follow-up to assess for cyst progression, implant stability, and patient symptoms.
- Operative treatment of isolated periprosthetic bone cysts without implant compromise consists of cyst debridement and grafting, whereas treatments for unstable implants in the setting of bone cysts include revision total ankle arthroplasty and arthrodesis.

INTRODUCTION

End-stage ankle arthritis is a debilitating condition that results in pain, loss of function, and an impaired quality of life.[1] The 2 major surgical treatment options to address this condition include tibiotalar arthrodesis and total ankle arthroplasty (TAA). TAA was introduced in the 1970s with the goal of providing pain relief while preserving range of motion to maintain optimal function. Unfortunately, initial attempts at TAA resulted in poor outcomes with high rates of failure including implant loosening and subsidence.[2,3] Given the poor outcomes of early-generation TAA, tibiotalar arthrodesis became the gold standard treatment of end-stage ankle arthritis. However, concerns regarding adjacent joint degeneration and altered gait mechanics following arthrodesis have led to an increasing interest in the optimization of TAA.[4–9] Modern advancements in implant design and surgical technique have demonstrated improved outcomes after TAA with comparable results to tibiotalar arthrodesis.[10–12] These improvements have resulted in a large increase in the number of TAAs being performed, especially when compared with tibiotalar arthrodesis.[13,14]

Despite improvements with TAA, postoperative complications requiring revision surgery remains a clinical problem. Hauer and colleagues[15] investigated revision rates after TAA by analyzing 43 clinical studies including 5806 primary TAAs and found a 7-year revision rate of 12.6%. In this study, implant loosening and subsidence was the cause of 49% of the revision TAAs. The formation of periprosthetic bone cysts is a common radiographic finding and can be a contributing factor to implant loosening and subsidence. The reported prevalence of periprosthetic bone cysts formation after TAA has been variable, but can be as high as 81% at an average follow-up of 44.6 months.[16] Along with implant loosening and subsidence, periprosthetic bone cysts can result in persistent pain and periprosthetic fracture. With the

---

Department of Orthopedic Surgery, Rush University Medical Center, 1611 W. Harrison Street, Suite 400, Chicago, IL 60612, USA
* Corresponding author.
E-mail address: danielbohl@gmail.com

Orthop Clin N Am 54 (2023) 109–119
https://doi.org/10.1016/j.ocl.2022.08.003
0030-5898/23/© 2022 Elsevier Inc. All rights reserved.

increasing volume of patients having undergone TAA, it is crucial for providers to understand the cause, proper evaluation, and subsequent management when periprosthetic bone cysts are encountered following TAA.

CAUSE

The cause of periprosthetic bone cysts after TAA is not entirely understood. The most commonly described process of periprosthetic bone cyst formation is osteolysis secondary to polyethylene (PE) wear, as has been seen with total hip and total knee arthroplasties.[17] Phagocytosis of debris from PE wear by macrophages can stimulate the release of cytokines resulting in the activation of osteoclasts causing bone resorption and cyst formation.[18,19] The rate of PE wear can be affected by the type of PE implanted. The use of conventional PE may produce increased wear particles when compared with highly cross-linked PE.[20,21] In addition, implant design may contribute to PE wear. The 2 major implant designs are a 3-component mobile-bearing prosthesis and a 2-component fixed-bearing prosthesis. The concern with a mobile-bearing prosthesis is the possibility of increased PE wear given 2 bearing surfaces and risk of PE subluxation resulting in edge loading. Assal and colleagues[22] compared reoperation rates between mobile-bearing and fixed-bearing implants at 3 years and found higher rates of reoperation with mobile-bearing implants. Specifically, mobile-bearing implants had higher rates of reoperations attributed to PE wear and cyst formation when compared with the fixed-bearing group. Similar findings of increased periprosthetic bone cysts with mobile-bearing implants have been observed in other studies as well.[23–25]

Although PE wear is a commonly reported cause for periprosthetic bone cyst formation, histologic evaluation of cystic tissue is conflicting. Schipper and colleagues[26] analyzed 57 pathology samples from areas of osteolysis after TAA and found large quantities of PE particles in osteolytic tissue. However, Gross and colleagues[27] found PE debris in only 7 of the 26 tissue samples taken from periprosthetic cysts with other findings including chronic inflammation, calcium pyrophosphate dehydrate crystals, unspecified foreign body reaction, ganglion cyst material, metal histiocytosis, and granulomatous reactions. These findings are similar to those of other studies with mixed histologic results, which may represent other causes of periprosthetic bone cysts.[28,29] Last, histologic analysis has identified hydroxyapatite as a contributing factor.[29,30]

In addition to PE wear, other explanations for the formation of periprosthetic bone cysts have been described. Micromotion between the bone and implant may contribute to cyst formation, and 1 factor contributing to increased micromotion is component malalignment.[31,32] In addition, component malalignment may increase PE wear in TAA due to increase in joint contact forces.[33,34] Lintz and colleagues[16] performed a retrospective review of patients with weight-bearing computed tomographic (CT) images following TAA and found that patients with residual hindfoot malalignment had an increased volume of periprosthetic cysts. With concerns regarding component malalignment, there is an increased focus on accurate and reliable positioning of components using patient-specific instrumentation (PSI). Escudero and colleagues[35] compared 51 patients undergoing TAA using PSI with 16 patients undergoing TAA using standard techniques and found no difference in osteolysis rates on plain radiographs at 2-year follow-up.[35] However, it is important to consider that PSI may not be superior to standard referencing techniques for component positioning.[36,37] Furthermore, there is some concern regarding the use of PSI increasing the risk of osteolysis secondary to greater soft tissue stripping, which may lead to ischemic necrosis and cyst formation.[35] If this is true, surgical approach may be a factor in osteolysis; however, to our knowledge this has not been evaluated.

In addition, patient factors may increase the risk of periprosthetic bone cyst formation including age, activity level, body mass, and even differences in cellular response to implant wear particles.[19] Lee and colleagues[38] evaluated if preoperative bone density of distal tibia and talus was associated with periprosthetic osteolysis following TAA, but found no association. Similarly, Cho and colleagues[39] found no difference in implant loosening between patients with rheumatoid arthritis and end-stage osteoarthritis after TAA. Additional research is required to determine patient risk factors for periprosthetic bone cyst formation.

Ultimately, the cause of periprosthetic bone cysts after TAA is not well understood and is likely multifactorial in nature. Other explanations are related to stress shielding,[40] implant material science,[41] high synovial fluid pressures,[42] and presence of preexisting cysts.[43] Further investigations are required to better understand the development of periprosthetic bone cysts, identification of risk factors, optimal implant design, ideal surgical technique, and subsequent prevention of this complication.

PATIENT EVALUATION OVERVIEW

Evaluation of patients with a painful TAA has been described previously.[44,45] First, a detailed history should be obtained. Questions regarding startup pain should be asked because this is often the first symptom of a problematic periprosthetic bone cyst. Other questions regarding trauma, infection, and other causes of pain should be asked to rule out other causes of symptoms. A thorough physical examination should be performed, and evidence of a ballooning bone cyst may be evident upon inspection and palpation (Fig. 1). Laboratory studies should be ordered to rule out infection.

In addition to history and physical examination, plain radiographs of the ankle should be obtained and detailed inspection of these radiographs should be performed to detect periprosthetic bone cysts, which is often defined as a radiolucent lesion measuring greater than 2 mm.[25] Radiographs should be compared with previous films to evaluate for interval change such as cyst progression, periprosthetic fracture, implant loosening, or subsidence (Fig. 2). In addition, Besse and colleagues[46] described 10 zones to classify the location of bone cyst formation with zones 1 to 5 viewed on the anteroposterior radiograph and zones 6 to 10 on the lateral radiograph. The clinical relevance of this classification system is not known but has been used in other investigations.[47,48]

Advanced imaging is useful for further evaluation of periprosthetic bone cysts. Specifically, CT imaging is more accurate at cyst detection and allows for volumetric assessment of these lesions when compared with plain radiographs.[47,48] In addition, weight-bearing CT may provide additional information regarding implant position and malalignment that may need to be corrected.[16] MRI is often limited in the setting of TAA given artifact from implants; however, metal artifact reduction sequencing can improve imaging quality and provide information regarding osteolytic cysts and bony edema.[49] Finally, nuclear medicine imaging can be obtained such as single-photon emission CT to assess biologic activity at the bone cyst and bone-implant interface. However, these findings can be nonspecific because increased activity may be seen in osteolysis, component loosening, infections, stress fractures, or a normal response in the early postoperative period.[50]

MANAGEMENT

Nonoperative Treatment

Nonoperative treatment is reserved for patients found to have small periprosthetic bone cysts without any symptoms. Although the presence of periprosthetic bone cysts can be common, patients are often asymptomatic.[51] These patients should be followed with clinical observation and evaluated for development of symptoms such as startup pain. Routine

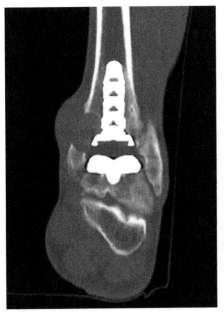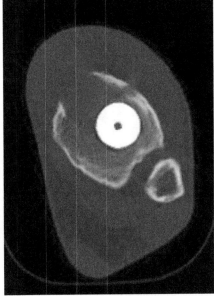

Fig. 1. Coronal and axial CT images representing a ballooning periprosthetic bone cyst of the medial malleolus that was evident on physical examination 5 years after TAA.

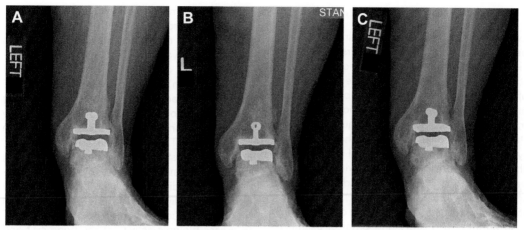

Fig. 2. (A) Anteroposterior radiograph of the left ankle 7 years after TAA. Progressive cyst formation can be seen inferior to the lateral aspect of the talar component at (B) 8 years and (C) 9 years postoperatively. (*Images courtesy of Dr. James W. Brodsky.*)

radiographs of the ankle should be obtained on an annual basis to assess for cyst progression, implant loosening, component subsidence, or impending fracture (Fig. 3). Advanced imaging should be obtained if any concerns are found on history, physical examination, or plain radiographs. Patients should be counseled regarding monitoring and instructed to return for repeat evaluation if symptoms develop.

Bone Cyst Debridement and Grafting

The primary surgical treatment of isolated bone cysts without implant compromise is cyst debridement with grafting. Indications to pursue surgical treatment in the setting of stable implants include large cysts, progressive increase in cyst size, and symptomatic cysts. Thresholds for surgical treatment regarding cyst size have been suggested as cysts greater than 10 mm,[27,52] but minimal evidence exists to

support this cutoff. The goal of cyst debridement and grafting is elimination of the cyst to relieve pain, provide implant stability, and prevent implant loosening or subsidence in the future.

Outcomes regarding cyst debridement and grafting have been variable. Yang and colleagues[53] reported promising results with this procedure by reviewing 210 consecutive mobile-bearing TAA where 19 cases (9%) required reoperation with cyst debridement, grafting, and PE liner exchange. This was the most common reoperation procedure observed, and they found no further progression of any of the lesions after the grafting procedure. In addition, Naude and colleagues[29] reported outcomes of cyst debridement, bone grafting, and PE liner exchange of 9 cystic lesions in 8 patients measuring at least 1.75 cm^3 on CT scan. The investigators demonstrated that 8 of the 9 lesions had successful graft incorporation when

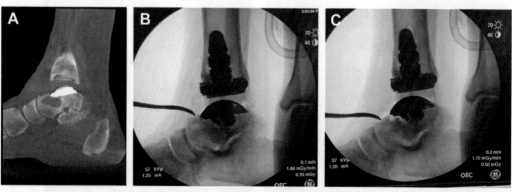

Fig. 3. (A) Sagittal CT imaging demonstrating periprosthetic bone cyst within the talar neck 7 years following TAA. (B and C) Intraoperative fluoroscopy demonstrating subsequent periprosthetic fracture of the talus and implant loosening.

evaluated postoperatively on CT at an average follow-up of 3 years. Last, Gross and colleagues[27] analyzed a total of 726 primary TAAs and reported outcomes of 31 patients who underwent bone cyst debridement and grafting. Failure of this procedure was defined as conversion to an arthrodesis or requiring future component revision. In this series, 27 (87%) patients had a successful outcome with 4 patients requiring arthrodesis or component revision, although 1 patient in the successful cohort did require a repeat bone grafting procedure. The investigators also use bisphosphonates for cysts greater than 10 mm.[27]

In contrast, Besse and colleagues[54] reported isolated cyst debridement and grafting in 14 patients who underwent TAA with poor results including a radiographic failure of 92% and need for arthrodesis in 28% of patients at an average of 34 weeks following grafting. Similarly, Kohonen and colleagues[52] performed a retrospective review of 65 periprosthetic bone cysts in 34 cases of TAA that underwent reoperation with cyst debridement and grafting.[52] The investigators found that 68% of the grafted lesions demonstrated continued progression of the cyst on postoperative CT with only 28% demonstrating radiographic success at an average follow-up of 3.8 years. One possible explanation for these conflicting findings between studies may be related to the specific TAA implant. Most of patients in these 2 studies had primary TAA with an implant that was discontinued due to high rates of early osteolysis, which may have an impact on the success of grafting procedures.

Additional considerations for patients undergoing cyst debridement and grafting include graft choice, role of PE exchange, assessment for possible cause of cyst formation, and optimal surgical technique. A variety of grafts have been used including autograft, allograft, supplementation with biologics, and use of bone cement; however, it is not clear what the optimal choice is. Also, concomitant PE liner exchange has been recommended at the time of cyst debridement and grafting given concerns of PE wear contributing to cyst formation.[29] However, Kohonen and colleagues[52] found no difference in cyst progression in those who underwent cyst grafting with or without PE exchange. Furthermore, patients should be assessed for component malposition and hindfoot malalignment because these may need to be addressed to reduce PE wear and implant micromotion. Finally, technical differences exist regarding this procedure. Lundeen and colleagues[55] described an endoscopic-assisted technique for cyst debridement and grafting. The investigators advocate for this method due to improved visualization of the cyst and superior debridement of cystic material, but this has not been proven.

In conclusion, the optimal management of periprosthetic bone cysts without implant compromise is not known. Cyst debridement and grafting appears to be a reasonable option for large cysts, progressive cysts, or painful cysts. Outcomes of this procedure are variable in terms of long-term radiographic success and avoidance of future arthrodesis or TAA component revision. However, treatment alternatives include nonoperative treatment with risk of further cyst progression and catastrophic implant failure in the future. In addition, revision TAA or conversion to arthrodesis can be performed instead, but these larger surgical procedures can be difficult to justify in an asymptomatic patient with stable implants. Further research is required to determine the success of this procedure and optimal techniques.

Revision Arthroplasty

Periprosthetic bone cysts may ultimately affect the integrity of a TAA prothesis causing implant loosening or component subsidence. In these clinic situations, revision of the tibial, talar, or all components is a potential treatment option. Large periprosthetic cysts remains a challenge during revision TAA because significant bone loss can limit the ability to revise either component. However, with the addition of revision TAA systems and modern primary TAA using minimal bone resection, revision TAA can a feasible surgical option.

With regard to the tibial component, adequate medial and lateral osseous structural support is needed, and standard tibial components often rely on a minimum of 50% osseous coverage at the distal tibia for fixation.[56,57] For large osseous defects of the distal tibia, implants with an intramedullary stem or custom tibial implants may be required to provide adequate fixation.[57–59] Bone defects should be addressed with techniques such as impaction grafting to improve the structural support for the implant and limit the possibility of periprosthetic cyst development following revision TAA.[57,59] Although grafting of bone defects can be performed at the time of revision TAA, some advocate for a staged procedure in which bone defects are first grafted followed by revision TAA approximately 3 to 4 months later.[60] Last, large PE liners can be used to help accommodate for a loss of distal tibial height.[57]

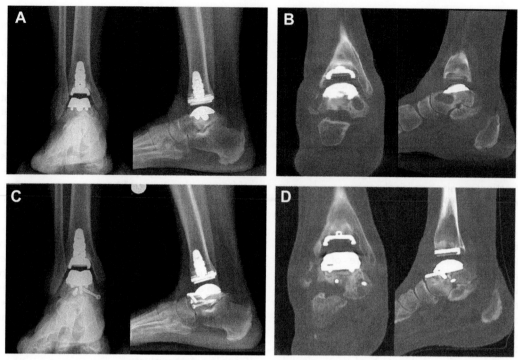

Fig. 4. (A) Preoperative radiographs and (B) CT images of a patient with recurrent right ankle pain 7 years after TAA demonstrating periprosthetic cysts of the talus. A periprosthetic talus fracture through the bone cyst and unstable talar component was seen intraoperatively (see Fig. 2). (C) Postoperative radiographs and (D) CT images 19 months after staged talar component explanation, cyst debridement, iliac crest bone grafting, and talar neck open reduction internal fixation followed by revision of the talar component 2 months later.

Periprosthetic cysts of the talus resulting in talar subsidence is a common cause for revision TAA.[61,62] Bone defects can be addressed in several ways for talar component revision. Grafting of bone defects and use of a revision talar component may be a viable option for small cysts or in cases of minimal subsidence (Fig. 4). The use of custom long-stemmed talar implants has been reported to improve fixation in the setting of greater bone loss and implant subsidence.[61,63] If the talus is unable to be salvaged, the use of a custom total talus implant in conjunction with a TAA may be a viable option for severe talar bone loss.[64–66]

Outcomes following revision TAA can be difficult to interpret in the setting of periprosthetic bone cysts because most studies contain small sample sizes or heterogeneous indications for revision. Behrens and colleagues[67] performed a retrospective review of 18 patients who underwent revision TAA for aseptic implant loosening or talar subsidence. Four patients (22.2%) required additional component revision at an average follow-up of 57.3 months, one of whom was for infection. Despite progression of osteolysis in 27.8% of patients following revision

TAA, patient-reported outcomes (PROs) remained comparable to primary TAA with similar implants. Lachman and colleagues[68] reviewed a larger cohort of 52 patients who underwent revision TAA for aseptic causes at an average of 5.5 years following primary TAA. Eleven patients (21.2%) required additional surgery with 6 converting to arthrodesis and the remaining 5 undergoing a second revision surgery. Otherwise, PROs improved following revision TAA but not to the level after primary TAA.

A larger series evaluating outcomes of revision TAA was published by Hintermann and colleagues[69] who reported a series of 117 revision TAAs with indications including implant loosening, subsidence, malposition, cyst formation, instability, and infection. At an average follow-up of 6.2 years following revision TAA, 17 patients (15%) required additional revision of components or arthrodesis. The remaining 100 patients demonstrated improvement in PROs with 81 patients obtaining good or excellent American Orthopedic Foot and Ankle Society hindfoot scores. The investigators deemed revision TAA as a viable treatment option for failure of primary TAA. Last, Egglestone and colleagues[70] performed a retrospective review of 31 cases of failed TAA undergoing surgical treatment with 21 proceeding with a revision TAA and 10 converting to arthrodesis. Patients undergoing revision TAA had superior PROs with an 87% implant survival at 4 years and arthrodesis was found to have a 20% nonunion rate.

The results of revision TAA may not be as promising as that of primary TAA[71]; however, it remains a viable option for patients with periprosthetic bone cysts that cause implant loosening or subsidence, especially if they desire to maintain range of motion and avoid the potential disadvantages of an arthrodesis.[69,72]

Arthrodesis

Massive expansion of periprosthetic bone cysts may cause dramatic bone loss and component subsidence, which can severely compromise the ability to perform a revision TAA. In addition, patients may fail multiple attempts at revision TAA resulting in soft tissue compromise, which further contributes to clinical decision making. In these scenarios, arthrodesis is the treatment of choice. Kotnis and colleagues[73] evaluated 14 patients undergoing surgical treatment of TAA aseptic loosening of which 5 patients underwent revision TAA and 9 proceeded with hindfoot arthrodesis. One of the revision TAAs required conversion to arthrodesis and another had evidence of radiographic failure, but declined surgery. Also, a higher proportion of patients undergoing revision TAA had persistent pain postoperatively compared with the hindfoot arthrodesis cohort. With these results, the investigators recommend arthrodesis as the preferred method for management of the failed TAA.

However, arthrodesis following failed TAA should not be viewed the same as a primary arthrodesis with longer time to union and inferior PROs related to pain and function.[74] In addition to bone loss, poor bone quality making rigid fixation difficult and compromise of the surrounding soft tissues creates a challenge for conversion of the failed TAA to an arthrodesis.[45] Union rates following arthrodesis for failed TAA have been variable with rates ranging from 58% to 95%.[75–82] Varying surgical techniques, patient factors, graft choice, and severity of bone loss likely contributes to the wide range of reported union rates. Gross and colleagues[83] performed a systematic review including 16 studies to determine the outcomes following conversion of a failed TAA to arthrodesis. A total of 193 patients were included, and an 84% union rate was observed after first attempts at

arthrodesis with improved union rates seen with isolated tibiotalar arthrodesis compared with tibiotalocalcaneal (TTC) arthrodesis.

When possible, a tibiotalar arthrodesis should be performed to preserve the motion of the subtalar joint. In addition, TTC arthrodesis after failed TAA appears to have inferior union rates when compared with isolated tibiotalar arthrodesis.[78,83] However, TTC arthrodesis may be indicated in the setting of severe talar bone loss limiting adequate fixation, severe talar subsidence involving the subtalar joint, or symptomatic subtalar arthritis.[84]

To address issues with bone loss and union during arthrodesis, graft is often required with options including autograft, allograft, and metal cage implants. Autograft can be used for smaller bone defects without need for significant structural support, although these patients may be better suited with attempted revision TAA. When bone loss is greater than 2 cm, a graft that provides structural support is necessary.[45] The most common allograft used in this scenario is a bulk femoral head allograft, which provides adequate bone stock and structural support for arthrodesis (Fig. 5). Coetzee and colleagues[85] reviewed outcomes of 45 cases of failed TAAs undergoing tibiotalar and TTC arthrodesis using femoral head allograft with an average of

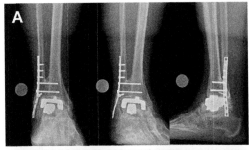

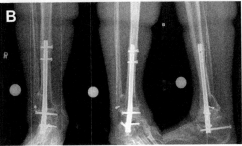

Fig. 5. (A) Weight-bearing radiographs 12 years following a right TAA in a patient with increasing right ankle pain demonstrating periprosthetic cyst formation involving the tibia and talus and with talar component subsidence. (B) Postoperative radiographs following conversion to a TTC arthrodesis with use of a femoral head allograft.

42.8 months follow-up. All 15 patients who underwent tibiotalar arthrodesis achieved union with high patient satisfaction. However, 5 (17%) of the 30 patients in the TTC arthrodesis group experienced nonunion.

In addition to bulk femoral head allograft, metal cage implants can be used to assist in the management of severe bone loss.[86] Potential advantages of these implants include customization to the specific patient and lower risk of collapse with improved mechanical properties.[87] Steele and colleagues[87] compared outcomes of patients who underwent TTC arthrodesis with either a femoral head allograft or a custom spherical implant. Eight patients underwent arthrodesis with a custom spherical implant, and 7 patients received a femoral head allograft. The spherical implant cohort had significantly higher rates of successful union and less graft resorption when compared with femoral head allograft. It is important to note that these procedures were not exclusively performed in patients with failed TAA. When looking at the use of metal cage implants specifically for failed TAA, outcomes are not as encouraging.[88] Aubret and colleagues[89] investigated union rates in 10 patients who underwent arthrodesis using a noncustom Trabecular Metal (Zimmer Biomet, Warsaw, IN, USA) implant with the use of iliac crest autograft. One patient underwent isolated tibiotalar arthrodesis and achieved union. Nine patients underwent TTC arthrodesis with 7 achieving tibiotalar union (78%), 5 achieving subtalar union (56%), and a total of 4 patients who had union at both the tibiotalar and subtalar joint (44%). Three patients (33%) went on to revision surgery.

SUMMARY

Periprosthetic bone cysts are common following TAA. Cysts can range from small asymptomatic cyst to large cysts causing catastrophic failure of TAA. Further investigation is needed to better understand the cause, risk factors, prevention, and optimal surgical treatment of this condition.

CLINICS CARE POINTS

- Periprosthetic bone cysts after TAA are a common radiographic finding with a wide range of clinical consequences
- Patients with small, asymptomatic cysts and stable TAA implants can be monitored on an annual basis with assessment for

development of symptoms, progression of cysts size, periprosthetic fracture, or implant loosening or subsidence.

- Patients with large, progressive, or symptomatic cysts and stable implants can be treated with cyst debridement and grafting. However, the success of this procedure is variable.
- Patients with implant loosening or subsidence can be treated with revision TAA or salvage arthrodesis depending on the severity of bone loss and soft tissue compromise.

DISCLOSURE

The authors have nothing to disclose.

REFERENCES

1. Glazebrook M, Daniels T, Younger A, et al. Comparison of health-related quality of life between patients with end-stage ankle and hip arthrosis. J Bone Joint Surg Am 2008;90(3):499–505.
2. Cracchiolo A 3rd, Deorio JK. Design features of current total ankle replacements: implants and instrumentation. J Am Acad Orthop Surg 2008; 16(9):530–40.
3. Henne TD, Anderson JG. Total ankle arthroplasty: a historical perspective. Foot Ankle Clin 2002;7(4): 695–702.
4. Sanders AE, Kraszewski AP, Ellis SJ, et al. Differences in gait and stair ascent after total ankle arthroplasty and ankle arthrodesis. Foot Ankle Int 2021;42(3):347–55.
5. Singer S, Klejman S, Pinsker E, et al. Ankle arthroplasty and ankle arthrodesis: gait analysis compared with normal controls. J Bone Joint Surg Am 2013;95(24):e191, 191-110.
6. Thomas R, Daniels TR, Parker K. Gait analysis and functional outcomes following ankle arthrodesis for isolated ankle arthritis. J Bone Joint Surg Am 2006;88(3):526–35.
7. Coester LM, Saltzman CL, Leupold J, et al. Long-term results following ankle arthrodesis for post-traumatic arthritis. J Bone Joint Surg Am 2001; 83(2):219–28.
8. Fuchs S, Sandmann C, Skwara A, et al. Quality of life 20 years after arthrodesis of the ankle. A study of adjacent joints. J Bone Joint Surg Br 2003; 85(7):994–8.
9. Hendrickx RP, Stufkens SA, de Bruijn EE, et al. Medium- to long-term outcome of ankle arthrodesis. Foot Ankle Int 2011;32(10):940–7.
10. Haddad SL, Coetzee JC, Estok R, et al. Intermediate and long-term outcomes of total ankle

arthroplasty and ankle arthrodesis. A systematic review of the literature. J Bone Joint Surg Am 2007; 89(9):1899–905.

11. Kim HJ, Suh DH, Yang JH, et al. Total ankle arthroplasty versus ankle arthrodesis for the treatment of end-stage ankle arthritis: a meta-analysis of comparative studies. Int Orthop 2017;41(1):101–9.

12. Stavrakis AI, SooHoo NF. Trends in Complication Rates Following Ankle Arthrodesis and Total Ankle Replacement. J Bone Joint Surg Am 2016;98(17): 1453–8.

13. Pugely AJ, Lu X, Amendola A, et al. Trends in the use of total ankle replacement and ankle arthrodesis in the United States Medicare population. Foot Ankle Int 2014;35(3):207–15.

14. Vakhshori V, Sabour AF, Alluri RK, et al. Patient and practice trends in total ankle replacement and tibiotalar arthrodesis in the united states from 2007 to 2013. J Am Acad Orthop Surg 2019;27(2):e77–84.

15. Hauer G, Hofer R, Kessler M, et al. Revision rates after total ankle replacement: a comparison of clinical studies and arthroplasty registers. Foot Ankle Int 2022;43(2):176–85.

16. Lintz F, Mast J, Bernasconi A, et al. 3D, Weight-bearing topographical study of periprosthetic cysts and alignment in total ankle replacement. Foot Ankle Int 2020;41(1):1–9.

17. Mehta N, Serino J, Hur ES, et al. Pathogenesis, evaluation, and management of osteolysis following total ankle arthroplasty. Foot Ankle Int 2021;42(2):230–42.

18. Besse JL. Osteolytic cysts with total ankle replacement: frequency and causes? Foot Ankle Surg 2015;21(2):75–6.

19. Espinosa N, Klammer G, Wirth SH. Osteolysis in total ankle replacement: how does it work? Foot Ankle Clin 2017;22(2):267–75.

20. Schipper ON, Haddad SL, Fullam S, et al. Wear characteristics of conventional ultrahigh-molecular-weight polyethylene versus highly cross-linked polyethylene in total ankle arthroplasty. Foot Ankle Int 2018;39(11):1335–44.

21. Bischoff JE, Fryman JC, Parcell J, et al. Influence of crosslinking on the wear performance of polyethylene within total ankle arthroplasty. Foot Ankle Int 2015;36(4):369–76.

22. Assal M, Kutaish H, Acker A, et al. Three-year rates of reoperation and revision following mobile versus fixed-bearing total ankle arthroplasty: a cohort of 302 patients with 2 implants of similar design. J Bone Joint Surg Am 2021;103(22):2080–8.

23. Gaudot F, Colombier JA, Bonnin M, et al. A controlled, comparative study of a fixed-bearing versus mobile-bearing ankle arthroplasty. Foot Ankle Int 2014;35(2):131–40.

24. Nunley JA, Adams SB, Easley ME, et al. Prospective randomized trial comparing mobile-bearing and fixed-bearing total ankle replacement. Foot Ankle Int 2019;40(11):1239–48.

25. Arcangelo J, Guerra-Pinto F, Pinto A, et al. Periprosthetic bone cysts after total ankle replacement. A systematic review and meta-analysis. Foot Ankle Surg 2019;25(2):96–105.

26. Schipper ON, Haddad SL, Pytel P, et al. Histological analysis of early osteolysis in total ankle arthroplasty. Foot Ankle Int 2017;38(4):351–9.

27. Gross CE, Huh J, Green C, et al. Outcomes of bone grafting of bone cysts after total ankle arthroplasty. Foot Ankle Int 2016;37(2):157–64.

28. van Wijngaarden R, van der Plaat L, Nieuwe Weme RA, et al. Etiopathogenesis of osteolytic cysts associated with total ankle arthroplasty, a histological study. Foot Ankle Surg 2015;21(2):132–6.

29. Naude JJ, Saragas NP, Ferrao PNF. CT scan assessment and functional outcome of periprosthetic bone grafting after total ankle arthroplasty at medium-term follow-up. Foot Ankle Int 2022;43(5): 609–19.

30. Singh G, Reichard T, Hameister R, et al. Ballooning osteolysis in 71 failed total ankle arthroplasties. Acta Orthop 2016;87(4):401–5.

31. Sundfeldt M, Carlsson LV, Johansson CB, et al. Aseptic loosening, not only a question of wear: a review of different theories. Acta Orthop 2006; 77(2):177–97.

32. Mondal S, Ghosh R. Effects of implant orientation and implant material on tibia bone strain, implant-bone micromotion, contact pressure, and wear depth due to total ankle replacement. Proc Inst Mech Eng H 2019;233(3):318–31.

33. Espinosa N, Walti M, Favre P, et al. Misalignment of total ankle components can induce high joint contact pressures. J Bone Joint Surg Am 2010;92(5): 1179–87.

34. Fukuda T, Haddad SL, Ren Y, et al. Impact of talar component rotation on contact pressure after total ankle arthroplasty: a cadaveric study. Foot Ankle Int 2010;31(5):404–11.

35. Escudero MI, Symes M, Bemenderfer TB, et al. Does patient-specific instrumentation have a higher rate of early osteolysis than standard referencing techniques in total ankle arthroplasty? A radiographic analysis. Foot Ankle Spec 2020;13(1): 32–42.

36. Escudero MI, Le V, Bemenderfer TB, et al. Total ankle arthroplasty radiographic alignment comparison between patient-specific instrumentation and standard instrumentation. Foot Ankle Int 2021;42(7): 851–8.

37. Heisler L, Vach W, Katz G, et al. Patient-Specific Instrumentation vs standard referencing in total ankle arthroplasty: a comparison of the radiologic outcome. Foot Ankle Int 2022;43(6):741–9.

38. Lee GW, Seo HY, Jung DM, et al. Comparison of preoperative bone density in patients with and without periprosthetic osteolysis following total ankle arthroplasty. Foot Ankle Int 2021;42(5): 575–81.

39. Cho NH, Kim S, Kwon DJ, et al. The prevalence of hallux valgus and its association with foot pain and function in a rural Korean community. J Bone Joint Surg Br 2009;91(4):494–8.

40. Waizy H, Behrens BA, Radtke K, et al. Bone cyst formation after ankle arthroplasty may be caused by stress shielding. A numerical simulation of the strain adaptive bone remodelling. Foot (Edinb) 2017;33:14–9.

41. Kormi S, Kohonen I, Koivu H, et al. Low rate of peri-implant osteolysis in trabecular metal total ankle replacement on short- to midterm follow-up. Foot Ankle Int 2021;42(11):1431–8.

42. Aspenberg P, van der Vis H. Fluid pressure may cause periprosthetic osteolysis. Particles are not the only thing. Acta Orthop Scand 1998;69(1): 1–4.

43. Bonnin M, Gaudot F, Laurent JR, et al. The Salto total ankle arthroplasty: survivorship and analysis of failures at 7 to 11 years. Clin Orthop Relat Res 2011;469(1):225–36.

44. Henry JK, Rider C, Cody E, et al. Evaluating and managing the painful total ankle replacement. Foot Ankle Int 2021;42(10):1347–61.

45. Hsu AR, Haddad SL, Myerson MS. Evaluation and management of the painful total ankle arthroplasty. J Am Acad Orthop Surg 2015;23(5):272–82.

46. Besse JL, Brito N, Lienhart C. Clinical evaluation and radiographic assessment of bone lysis of the AES total ankle replacement. Foot Ankle Int 2009; 30(10):964–75.

47. Viste A, Al Zahrani N, Brito N, et al. Periprosthetic osteolysis after AES total ankle replacement: Conventional radiography versus CT-scan. Foot Ankle Surg 2015;21(3):164–70.

48. Kohonen I, Koivu H, Pudas T, et al. Does computed tomography add information on radiographic analysis in detecting periprosthetic osteolysis after total ankle arthroplasty? Foot Ankle Int 2013;34(2):180–8.

49. de Cesar Netto C, Fonseca LF, Fritz B, et al. Metal artifact reduction MRI of total ankle arthroplasty implants. Eur Radiol 2018;28(5):2216–27.

50. Serino J, Kunze KN, Jacobsen SK, et al. Nuclear medicine for the orthopedic foot and ankle surgeon. Foot Ankle Int 2020;41(5):612–23.

51. Yoon HS, Lee J, Choi WJ, et al. Periprosthetic osteolysis after total ankle arthroplasty. Foot Ankle Int 2014;35(1):14–21.

52. Kohonen I, Koivu H, Tiusanen H, et al. Are periprosthetic osteolytic lesions in ankle worth bone grafting? Foot Ankle Surg 2017;23(2):128–33.

53. Yang HY, Wang SH, Lee KB. The HINTEGRA total ankle arthroplasty: functional outcomes and implant survivorship in 210 osteoarthritic ankles at a mean of 6.4 years. Bone Joint J 2019;101-B(6): 695–701.

54. Besse JL, Lienhart C, Fessy MH. Outcomes following cyst curettage and bone grafting for the management of periprosthetic cystic evolution after AES total ankle replacement. Clin Podiatr Med Surg 2013;30(2):157–70.

55. Lundeen GA, Barousse PS, Moles LH, et al. Technique tip: endoscopic-assisted curettage and bone grafting of periprosthetic total ankle arthroplasty bone cysts. Foot Ankle Int 2021;42(2):224–9.

56. Myerson MS, Won HY. Primary and revision total ankle replacement using custom-designed prostheses. Foot Ankle Clin 2008;13(3):521–38, x.

57. Jonck JH, Myerson MS. Revision total ankle replacement. Foot Ankle Clin 2012;17(4):687–706.

58. Devries JG, Berlet GC, Lee TH, et al. Revision total ankle replacement: an early look at agility to INBONE. Foot Ankle Spec 2011;4(4):235–44.

59. Gaden MT, Ollivere BJ. Periprosthetic aseptic osteolysis in total ankle replacement: cause and management. Clin Podiatr Med Surg 2013;30(2): 145–55.

60. Horisberger M, Henninger HB, Valderrabano V, et al. Bone augmentation for revision total ankle arthroplasty with large bone defects. Acta Orthop 2015;86(4):412–4.

61. Li SY, Myerson MS. Management of Talar component subsidence. Foot Ankle Clin 2017;22(2): 361–89.

62. Glazebrook MA, Arsenault K, Dunbar M. Evidence-based classification of complications in total ankle arthroplasty. Foot Ankle Int 2009;30(10):945–9.

63. Ketz J, Myerson M, Sanders R. The salvage of complex hindfoot problems with use of a custom talar total ankle prosthesis. J Bone Joint Surg Am 2012;94(13):1194–200.

64. Bejarano-Pineda L, DeOrio JK, Parekh SG. Combined total talus replacement and total ankle arthroplasty. J Surg Orthop Adv 2020;29(4):244–8.

65. Kurokawa H, Taniguchi A, Morita S, et al. Total ankle arthroplasty incorporating a total talar prosthesis: a comparative study against the standard total ankle arthroplasty. Bone Joint J 2019;101-B(4): 443–6.

66. Kanzaki N, Chinzei N, Yamamoto T, et al. Clinical outcomes of total ankle arthroplasty with total talar prosthesis. Foot Ankle Int 2019;40(8):948–54.

67. Behrens SB, Irwin TA, Bemenderfer TB, et al. Clinical and radiographic outcomes of revision total ankle arthroplasty using an intramedullary-referencing implant. Foot Ankle Int 2020;41(12): 1510–8.

68. Lachman JR, Ramos JA, Adams SB, et al. Revision surgery for metal component failure in total ankle arthroplasty. Foot Ankle Orthop 2019;4(1). 2473011418813026.

69. Hintermann B, Zwicky L, Knupp M, et al. HINTE-GRA revision arthroplasty for failed total ankle prostheses. J Bone Joint Surg Am 2013;95(13): 1166–74.

70. Egglestone A, Kakwani R, Aradhyula M, et al. Outcomes of revision surgery for failed total ankle replacement: revision arthroplasty versus arthrodesis. Int Orthop 2020;44(12):2727–34.

71. Lachman JR, Ramos JA, Adams SB, et al. Patient-reported outcomes before and after primary and revision total ankle arthroplasty. Foot Ankle Int 2019;40(1):34–41.

72. Hordyk PJ, Fuerbringer BA, Roukis TS. Sagittal ankle and midfoot range of motion before and after revision total ankle replacement: a retrospective comparative analysis. J Foot Ankle Surg 2018;57(3): 521–6.

73. Kotnis R, Pasapula C, Anwar F, et al. The management of failed ankle replacement. J Bone Joint Surg Br 2006;88(8):1039–47.

74. Rahm S, Klammer G, Benninger E, et al. Inferior results of salvage arthrodesis after failed ankle replacement compared to primary arthrodesis. Foot Ankle Int 2015;36(4):349–59.

75. Deleu PA, Devos Bevernage B, Maldague P, et al. Arthrodesis after failed total ankle replacement. Foot Ankle Int 2014;35(6):549–57.

76. Kamrad I, Henricson A, Magnusson H, et al. Outcome after salvage arthrodesis for failed total ankle replacement. Foot Ankle Int 2016;37(3): 255–61.

77. Culpan P, Le Strat V, Piriou P, et al. Arthrodesis after failed total ankle replacement. J Bone Joint Surg Br 2007;89(9):1178–83.

78. Berkowitz MJ, Clare MP, Walling AK, et al. Salvage of failed total ankle arthroplasty with fusion using structural allograft and internal fixation. Foot Ankle Int 2011;32(5):S493–502.

79. Hopgood P, Kumar R, Wood PL. Ankle arthrodesis for failed total ankle replacement. J Bone Joint Surg Br 2006;88(8):1032–8.

80. Kitaoka HB, Romness DW. Arthrodesis for failed ankle arthroplasty. J Arthroplasty 1992;7(3):277–84.

81. Carlsson AS, Montgomery F, Besjakov J. Arthrodesis of the ankle secondary to replacement. Foot Ankle Int 1998;19(4):240–5.

82. Ali AA, Forrester RA, O'Connor P, et al. Revision of failed total ankle arthroplasty to a hindfoot fusion: 23 consecutive cases using the Phoenix nail. Bone Joint J 2018;100-B(4):475–9.

83. Gross C, Erickson BJ, Adams SB, et al. Ankle arthrodesis after failed total ankle replacement: a systematic review of the literature. Foot Ankle Spec 2015;8(2):143–51.

84. Adams SB. Salvage Arthrodesis for Failed Total Ankle Replacement. Foot Ankle Clin 2020;25(2):281–91.

85. Coetzee JC, Den Hartog BD, Stone McGaver R, et al. Femoral Head Allografts for Talar Body Defects. Foot Ankle Int 2021;42(7):815–23.

86. Bullens P, de Waal Malefijt M, Louwerens JW. Conversion of failed ankle arthroplasty to an arthrodesis. Technique using an arthrodesis nail and a cage filled with morsellized bone graft. Foot Ankle Surg 2010;16(2):101–4.

87. Steele JR, Kadakia RJ, Cunningham DJ, et al. Comparison of 3D printed spherical implants versus femoral head allografts for tibiotalocalcaneal arthrodesis. J Foot Ankle Surg 2020;59(6):1167–70.

88. Carlsson A. Unsuccessful use of a titanium mesh cage in ankle arthrodesis: a report on three cases operated on due to a failed ankle replacement. J Foot Ankle Surg 2008;47(4):337–42.

89. Aubret S, Merlini L, Fessy M, et al. Poor outcomes of fusion with Trabecular Metal implants after failed total ankle replacement: early results in 11 patients. Orthop Traumatol Surg Res 2018;104(2):231–7.

Printed and bound by CPI Group (UK) Ltd, Croydon, CR0 4YY

08/05/2025

01864715-0011